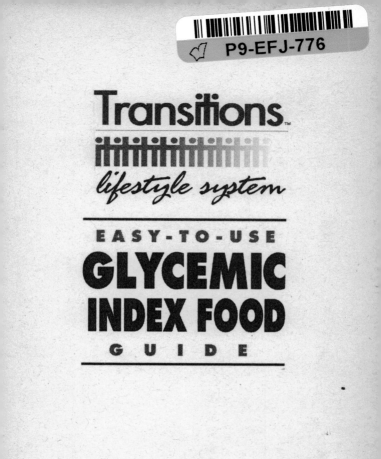

Transitions™

lifestyle system

EASY-TO-USE
GLYCEMIC
INDEX FOOD
GUIDE

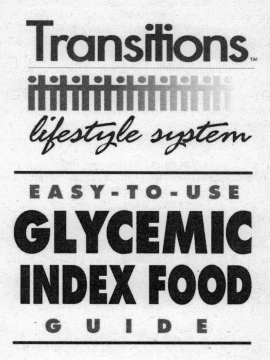

Transitions™

lifestyle system

EASY-TO-USE

GLYCEMIC INDEX FOOD

GUIDE

DR. SHARI LIEBERMAN

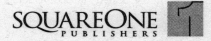

SQUAREONE
PUBLISHERS

The information and advice contained in this book are based upon the research and the personal and professional experiences of the author. They are not intended as a substitute for consulting with a health care professional. The publisher and author are not responsible for any adverse effects or consequences resulting from the use of any of the suggestions presented in this book. All matters pertaining to your physical health should be supervised by a health care professional. It is a sign of wisdom, not cowardice, to seek a second or third opinion.

COVER DESIGNER: Jeannie Tudor
IN-HOUSE EDITORS: Ariel Colletti, Marie Caratozzolo,
and Joanne Abrams
TYPESETTER: Gary A. Rosenberg

Square One Publishers
115 Herricks Road • Garden City Park, NY 11040
516-535-2010 • 877-900-BOOK
www.SquareOnePublishers.com

ISBN-10: 0-7570-0245-5
ISBN-13: 978-0-7570-0245-8

Printed in the United States of America

10   9   8   7   6   5   4

CONTENTS

The Glycemic Index Food Guide

*To every person who truly believes
that they can play a major role
in the improvement of their own health.*

ACKNOWLEDGMENTS

This book would not be possible without the commitment of JR, Loren, Marty, Dennis, and all my friends at Market America. Their vision and steadfast commitment to excellence is dramatically improving the health of this nation and the world.

I want to thank Joanne Abrams, Ariel Colletti, and Marie Caratozzolo, the editorial staff at Square One, for overseeing the work necessary to make this book both useful and accessible. Also I would like to thank typesetter Gary Rosenberg for his excellent layout and artist Jeannie Tudor for her lovely graphic designs. I would like to thank Rudy Shur, my publisher, for believing in my work and sharing my own vision of a healthier world.

INTRODUCTION

Originally designed as a guide for people with diabetes, the glycemic index is an important new nutritional tool that now has wide-ranging uses. By indicating how quickly a given food triggers a rise in blood sugar, it enables everyone—from diabetics, to individuals who want to lose weight, to people who simply want to remain healthy—to choose the foods that can help them meet their dietary and health goals. This book is an easy-to-use guide to the glycemic index, or GI. Whether you have been relying on the GI for years or have just heard about this wonderful tool, you're sure to find it invaluable as you learn about the GI and use it to make smart food choices.

The book begins by answering a number of frequently asked questions about the glycemic index. Here you'll get a crash course in carbohydrates, which is what the GI is all about; learn about the glycemic index itself; and discover the importance of the GI in preventing and managing a host of disorders, from diabetes to cancer to fatigue. If you've ever wondered why people with diabetes are urged to avoid certain foods, or simply why some foods so often lead to feelings of lethargy, you're sure to

1

enjoy this easy-to-read Q and A. This section also addresses some issues that often confuse people when they first glance at the glycemic index of different foods. Why are certain foods, like meat and fish, not ranked on the glycemic index? Does eating more of a food cause its GI number to increase? What is glycemic load, or GL? Since carrots have a high GI, does that mean that they're an unhealthy food? Perhaps most important, the Q and A tells you how to use the glycemic index to create a diet that not only is healthy but also includes the foods you love. The fact is that you don't have to give up your favorite foods—not even if they rank high on the index. You just have to learn to integrate them wisely in your diet by balancing high-GI choices with low-GI foods.

After the Q and A section, you'll find the heart of the book: The Glycemic Index Food Guide. This table presents an alphabetical listing of hundreds of common foods and beverages, including many combination and prepared foods, along with their glycemic index ranking and their glycemic load. If you've already used other GI lists, you'll immediately see that this one is different. First, while many lists express portion size in grams, this one has converted grams to familiar ounce measurements. Second, while other lists force you to search endlessly for a particular food, this one places each food not only under its name, but also under logical categories. Say you're looking for udon noodles, for instance. Whether you search for it under "Udon,"

"Asian Foods," or just plain "Pasta," you'll quickly find its GI. In fact, several ethnic categories have been created to make it easy to dine at your favorite restaurant. You'll also see that instead of using confusing GI numbers, this guide clearly identifies the glycemic index of a food as being low, medium, or high, so that you immediately understand its effect on blood glucose levels. Meanwhile, intriguing questions and tips have been sprinkled throughout the guide, leading you to informative discussions and highlighting good food choices.

Because there's so much to learn about the glycemic index, and because more information is always becoming available, the book ends with a list of helpful websites. These sites provide more detailed information about topics of interest, and in many cases offer continuously updated databases of foods. Check them out, and you're sure to learn even more about this fascinating subject, as well as gleaning practical tips and suggestions for meeting your dietary goals.

Whether you are interested in controlling your glucose levels to manage a specific health problem, you're trying to boost your energy levels, you wish to achieve a healthier weight, or you simply want to enhance your overall well-being, this guide was designed to help you every step of the way. Turn the page, and learn how the glycemic index can change your life.

PART ONE

FREQUENTLY ASKED QUESTIONS ABOUT THE GLYCEMIC INDEX

FAQs
About the GI

This book is an easy-to-use guide to the glycemic index (GI) of various common foods and beverages. Whether you are interested in controlling your GI to manage your diabetes, lose weight, increase your heart health, boost your energy level, or simply improve your overall well-being, the table that begins on page 37 will help you do so. But if the concept of glycemic index is a new one for you, it makes sense to take a little time to learn about it. That's why this simple question-and-answer section was written. It will first introduce you to carbohydrates—the all-important nutrient that the glycemic index is all about. It will then help you understand the glycemic index itself, explaining exactly what it shows for each of the foods listed, and how it can be used when making dietary choices. Finally, it will take a brief look at some common health problems that are affected by GI and describe how these disorders can be better managed through use of the glycemic index.

7

UNDERSTANDING CARBOHYDRATES

What are carbohydrates?

Carbohydrates are one of the body's three sources of fuel, the other sources being protein and fat. All three of these sources contain calories, with carbs and protein supplying four calories per gram, and fat supplying nine calories per gram. When the body burns a calorie—whether from a carbohydrate, a protein, or a fat—energy is released. Carbohydrates, however, have the distinction of being the human body's main and most efficient source of energy.

Carbohydrates are manufactured by plants during the process of photosynthesis. Chemically, carbs are molecules formed by carbon, hydrogen, and oxygen. Animals, including humans, obtain carbohydrates by eating foods that contain them— plant-based foods such as potatoes, rice, bread, and so on. Meat, poultry, fish, and eggs contain negligible amounts of carbohydrates.

Are there different types of carbohydrates?

Carbohydrates are generally divided into two categories: simple carbohydrates and complex carbohydrates.

All carbohydrates consist of units of sugar known as saccharide units. Those carbs that contain only one, two, or three sugar units are known as *simple carbohydrates*, or *simple sugars*. These carbs, which include table sugar, are quickly broken down by the body to release energy.

Complex carbohydrates are chains of hundreds or even thousands of simple carbs that have been bonded together. These carbs are broken down by the body more slowly, providing a slow, steady release of energy.

Complex carbohydrates can be further broken down into two groups: digestible carbs (starch) and indigestible carbs (fiber). *Digestible carbohydrates* can be processed by the human digestive system and used for fuel. *Indigestible carbohydrates* cannot be absorbed by the human digestive system, although they do have many healthful benefits. All unprocessed fruits, vegetables, grains, beans, and nuts contain both digestible and indigestible forms of carbohydrate.

How are different carbohydrates metabolized by the body?

When a food containing complex carbohydrates—oatmeal, for instance—is eaten, its high fiber content prevents it from quickly leaving the stomach. This results in a feeling of fullness. The food then moves on to the small intestine, where the two types of complex carbohydrate—starch and fiber—separate from each other. The starch portion then pushes itself through the fiber and slowly makes it way towards the villi, which are the fingerlike projections of the small intestine that absorb nutrients. By this time, the starch has been broken down into glucose and is ready to be transported to the blood. When the glucose enters the blood, blood sugar levels rise. This, in turn, causes the pancreas to secrete insulin, a hormone that allows glucose to be transported to the cells. When glucose enters the cells, some of it is immediately used as fuel, some is stored in the muscles and liver as reserve fuel, and any remaining glucose is stored as fat. As glucose is distributed throughout the body, blood sugar levels begin to fall.

A very different scenario occurs when a food that contains simple carbohydrates is consumed— a sugar-sweetened soft drink or a square of fudge, for instance. Because this type of food has little or no fiber to slow its movement through the stomach, it is rapidly transported to the small intestine. Once there, without the fiber needed to cause more gradual absorption, the starch is quickly absorbed into the bloodstream, causing a surge of glucose in the blood and a resulting spike in blood sugar levels. Soon afterward, the pancreas, in response, releases a spike of insulin, which immediately begins the task of moving the glucose to cells located throughout the body.

What does this have to do with the glycemic index?

As you've seen, different types of carbohydrates are processed differently by the body, and consequently have different effects on blood glucose levels. The glycemic index, or GI, ranks carbohydrate-rich foods according to their effect on blood glucose levels.

UNDERSTANDING THE GLYCEMIC INDEX

What is the glycemic index?

Created by Dr. David J. Jenkins and a team of researchers at the University of Toronto in 1981, to help diabetes patients manage their blood sugar levels, the glycemic index (GI) is a ranking system for foods containing carbohydrates. The GI number signifies how quickly a food triggers a rise in blood glucose (sugar). The higher the number, the greater the response. Foods with a low GI ranking break down slowly during digestion, resulting in a gradual release of glucose into the bloodstream. Foods with high GI numbers, on the other hand, break down more quickly, causing an undesirable surge of blood glucose and a resulting surge of insulin.

Why is the glycemic index important?

As you will see in the section that begins on page 21, regular consumption of high-glycemic foods leads to a greater chance of developing a number of serious health problems, including insulin resistance, type II diabetes, obesity, cancer, and cardiovascular disease. A primarily low-glycemic diet is helpful in lowering blood cholesterol levels, controlling weight, maintaining energy, and promoting overall good health.

How is the glycemic index of a food calculated?

Foods are ranked on the glycemic index according to their ability to raise blood sugar levels after being ingested. To determine this, an amount of food that contains 50 grams of carbohydrate is fed to eight to ten people. Then, over the next two hours, the blood glucose levels of the test subjects are checked every fifteen to thirty minutes. The test is repeated two to three times, and the values are averaged and compared to a *standard* or *reference* food—usually pure glucose. Glucose has been given an arbitrary glycemic index value of 100. Foods with a GI number of 70 or more are considered high glycemic; those that fall between 56 and 69 are in the medium range; and those ranked 55 or less are considered low.

Why do certain foods within the same food group—such as potatoes and rice—have different rankings on the GI?

Certain foods, such as potatoes, rice, and oats, can have GI numbers that vary widely. There are a number of possible explanations for these value variations. Assorted types of potatoes, for instance, contain varying amounts of fiber. They (as well as different rice varieties) also contain different kinds of starch, which break down differently during digestion. For instance, a white potato provides a rapidly digestible starch *and* has virtually no fiber. The result is a high GI. But despite its name and its sweet taste, a sweet potato has a lower GI. Why? One reason is that it's rich in fiber. Other factors that create variations include where and how certain products are grown, as well as differences in manufacturing methods. Preparation techniques can also affect GI. (To learn more about this, see pages 19 to 20.)

People are often puzzled by the GI variations found among various fruits. While apples and bananas have low GI values, for instance, dates and watermelon are high-GI foods. Why? Again, various amounts of fiber are partly to blame, as are different sugars. The sugar fructose has a very low GI, for instance, so that high-fructose fruits tend to have a low GI, too. On the other hand, the sugar glucose has a high GI, so that fruits with more available glucose have a higher glycemic index value.

How is it possible that a plain baked potato has a higher GI value than potato chips?

Remember that the glycemic index number is an indication of the rate at which the carbohydrate is digested—the faster the digestion, the greater (and less desirable) the glucose response. The presence of fat in foods tends to slow down the rate of digestion, which, in turn, slows down the glucose response. However, this does not mean the food is a healthy choice. If the fat is saturated, it can increase the risk of health problems such as cardiovascular disease. Even a high intake of polyunsaturated fat can have adverse health consequences, such as obesity.

Why is pasta ranked as a low-glycemic food?

Interestingly, most pasta varieties, as well as a number of Asian noodles, have a fairly low GI. This is because the gluten (protein) network that is present in pasta dough traps the starch granules, causing them to be digested more slowly.

Why isn't sugar ranked high on the GI?

Prior to the creation of the glycemic index, scientists believed that sugar was digested very quickly and, thereby, produced a rapid increase in blood sugar levels. During GI testing, however, a surprising discovery was made. Although the body processes glucose very easily, it cannot easily metabolize fructose—a sugar (monosaccharide) found in fruits. For this reason, fructose has a GI of 23, which falls into the low range. Ordinary table sugar (sucrose) is a disaccharide made up of one molecule of glucose and one molecule of fructose. This gives sugar a GI of 65, placing it in the medium range.

Certain foods such as meat, fish, and even some vegetables are not ranked on the glycemic index. Why?

In the discussion of glycemic index testing, it was explained that all foods are tested by using the amount of that food which provides 50 grams of carbohydrate. For some foods—potatoes, for instance—that amount is a standard portion. But for other foods, huge amounts would have to be eaten before a test subject had ingested 50 grams. For instance, you would have to consume about twenty cups of cauliflower—five quarts!—to get the needed 50 grams of carbs. That's why only foods that contain significant amounts of carbohydrates are ranked on the glycemic index. In the table in this book, those foods that contain no carbs, or so few carbs that they can't be tested, are marked "Insignificant Carbs." When eaten by themselves, these foods are not likely to cause a significant rise in blood sugar. In addition to many vegetables, insignificant-carb foods include meat, fish, and poultry, as well as tofu, most nuts, avocados, cheese, eggs, and alcoholic beverages.

Be aware, though, that although standard portions of these foods are thought not to affect blood sugar levels, not all of them promote good health. While some insignificant-carb foods, such as leafy greens, are healthful and can be eaten all day; others, like red meat, are known to contain unhealthy amounts of saturated fat; and still others provide a high number of calories, which can contribute to weight gain. For this reason, it is important to keep in mind that the word "insignificant" refers to the food's effect on blood sugar levels only, and not to its total impact on your health.

Why don't alcoholic beverages have GI numbers? Aren't they made from high-carbohydrate ingredients?

Most alcoholic beverages—liquor, wine, and beer—contain no (or very few) carbohydrates. Although various "hard" liquors, such as scotch, gin, and vodka, are made from high-carbohydrate ingredients, like sugar, potatoes, and grains, they contain zero carbs. This is due to the fermentation and distillation process. For wine, most of the sugar found in grapes (carbs) is also converted to alcohol during the wine-making process, but a very small amount of residual sugar remains. When beer is fermented during the brewing process, the sugar (maltose) it contains is consumed by yeast and converted to alcohol. The resulting beer contains a small number of carbohydrates—about 3 grams per 100 milliliters, which is a fraction of the amount contained in an equal serving of most soft drinks.

It is important to keep in mind that although alcoholic beverages are practically carb free, they are *all* high in calories. Alcohol itself contains 7 calories per gram! This is higher than the amount found in protein and carbohydrates (about 4 calories per gram), and nearly as much as the amount contained in fat (about 9 calories per gram). This means that an excessive consumption of alcoholic beverages is likely to pack on the pounds.

Diabetics, in particular, should not be seduced by alcohol's insignificant-carb status. If you have diabetes and take insulin shots or oral diabetes pills, you risk low blood sugar every time you drink alcohol. In fact, drinking as little as two ounces of alcohol on an empty stomach—about two drinks—can lead to very low blood sugar levels. The truth is that alcohol consumption can result in low blood sugar in *anyone*—not just diabetics. And all too commonly, this causes fatigue and resulting cravings for sweet high-GI foods.

Does eating more of a food cause its GI number to increase?

No. The GI number indicates its *ranking* compared with other foods containing the same amount of carbohydrates. This number, therefore, always stays the same. If, however, you eat increased amounts of a food containing carbohydrates, the resulting blood glucose response will be higher. That's what the glycemic load, discussed below, is all about.

What is glycemic load?

When determining true blood glucose levels, the GI value (*quality*) of the carbohydrate in a food is only one of two factors that must be considered. The other is the amount (*quantity*) of that carbohydrate being consumed. That's why scientists came up with the glycemic load (GL). The GL reflects not only the glycemic index of a food, but also the amount of carbohydrates ingested.

The GL of a food is determined through a simple mathematical formula. The food's GI number is multiplied by the number of carbohydrates (in grams) contained in a given portion of that food, and then divided by 100.

glycemic index number x number of
carbohydrate grams ÷ 100 = glycemic load

Each number of the GL is equivalent to 1 gram of carbohydrate from pure glucose. The lower the GL number, the better. A number of 20 or more is considered high; a number between 11 and 19 falls in the medium range; a number of 10 or less is considered low. A daily GL of 80 or less is regarded as low, while a GL of 120 or more is considered high.

Why is glycemic load so important?

Glycemic load puts the GI in perspective and helps explain some GI ratings that would otherwise be misleading. Let's look at carrots, for example. Raw carrots are considered a high-GI food. However, carrots are relatively low in carbohydrates, so to eat the 50 grams of carbohydrates that test subjects must consume in order to calculate GI, you would have to eat nearly three cups of carrots. Since most people eat less than this at a sitting, probably stopping at a cup, the glycemic load of carrots is quite low. By taking into account not just the glycemic index but also serving size, the GL gives you a more realistic picture of how the food you are eating is likely to affect your blood glucose level.

Do I have to give up my favorite high-GI foods?

No, you just have to integrate them into your diet wisely. First, exercise portion control so that you eat less. Then, rather than eating that food on an empty stomach, have it after a meal. For instance, if you eat a high-GI food like watermelon after dinner, the food you ate at dinner will slow the absorption of the watermelon and prevent a spike in your body's glucose response. When choosing items like bread or potatoes (of which there are various types that range in rankings on the GI), opt for the lower-glycemic varieties of those foods. For example, choose cracked or sprouted whole wheat bread—bread with 3 to 4 grams of fiber per slice or that's labelled "low net carb"—over white bread or most commercial wheat breads. Select coarse oatmeal or porridge over instant varieties. And choose pasta over rice. When eating a less-desirable high-gly-cemic food during a meal, be sure to balance it with some low-glycemic choices.

What factors can affect the GI of a food, making it higher or lower than shown on GI tables?

Although the table that begins on page 37 may indicate that a food has a low, medium, or high GI, various factors can affect its GI, making it higher or lower by the time it reaches your table. That's why it pays to be aware of the following:

❏ The ripening process affects a food's GI. As a fruit or vegetable becomes riper, its sugar content rises and its GI becomes higher.

❏ Processing a food generally makes its GI higher. A mashed potato has a higher GI than a baked potato, although both are in the high range; a glass of orange juice usually has a higher GI than a whole orange; processed (finely ground) whole wheat bread has a higher GI than stone-ground whole wheat bread. Why? Because processing makes a food quicker and easier to digest.

❑ Cooking a food generally makes its GI higher. Pasta that's cooked for twenty minutes has a higher GI than pasta that's cooked for ten minutes, for instance. This is because cooking, like processing, hastens the eventual digestion of a food. Just be aware that if the cooking process adds fat to the food, it will actually *lower* the food's GI. That's why potato chips have a lower GI than baked potatoes.

Finally, because meals usually combine more than one food, keep in mind that everything you eat along with a given food will affect its glycemic index. The GI of a meal can be estimated by averaging the GIs of the individual foods while taking into account the relative amounts eaten. In other words, a large portion is likely to have a more significant effect than a small portion. Remember that the best way to lower the GI of a meal is to eat more fiber. While the addition of protein and fat will lower GI, too, it can also cause a host of health problems.

Can I estimate the GI of a packaged food that isn't included in the table?

In many cases, you can. First, look at the ingredient label. If the first few ingredients listed are low GI foods like chicken and lentils, you can consider it to have a relatively low GI. Second, some packages list *net carbs.* Also called *digestible carbs,* the term net carbs refers to the total carbohydrates in a food that can be absorbed and digested—the amount that will affect blood sugar levels. A snack with net carbs of 5 would have a low GI. A meal with 10 to 15 net carbs would have a low to moderate GI. Finally, if net carbs aren't listed, you can determine the food's net carbs by subtracting the grams of fiber, sugar alcohols, fructose, and glycerine from the total carbohydrate content. Some packages list the amounts of each of these substances, and some do not. When the amounts aren't listed, you should be able to obtain this information from the manufacturer.

HEALTH DISORDERS ASSOCIATED WITH THE GLYCEMIC INDEX

How are high-GI foods associated with diabetes?

When the body is fed simple carbohydrates year after year in the form of refined foods such as white sugar, white bread, sugary soft drinks, and the like, a condition known as *insulin resistance* can develop. In this condition, the cells no longer respond properly to insulin, and refuse to let the insulin transport glucose to the cells. To compensate, the body secretes even more insulin into the bloodstream in an effort to reduce blood glucose levels. But because the cells are unable to respond to the insulin, both insulin levels and blood sugar levels remain chronically high. At this point, insulin resistance can spiral into type II diabetes. Also called *adult onset diabetes* and *non-insulin-dependent diabetes*, *type II diabetes*—a disorder in which the body's cells fail to take up glucose from the bloodstream—is a chronic progressive disease that accounts for about 90 percent of all diabetics.

Researchers have found that the development of type II diabetes is strongly associated with the consumption of high-GI foods. In the Harvard Nurses' Health Study of 80,000 women, those who ate greater amounts of higher-GI refined carbohydrates had a two-and-a-half times greater risk of developing type II diabetes than those who ate a diet rich in lower-glycemic index whole grains, fruits, and vegetables.

How are high-GI foods associated with obesity?

Researchers have shown that the consumption of high-GI foods tends to increase hunger and promote overeating, which can then lead to excess weight gain and obesity. You've already learned about one way in which this occurs. High-fiber foods, which generally have a low GI, move slowly through the body. Because they stay in the stomach for a relatively long period of time, they promote a feeling of fullness. On the other hand, high-GI foods, which generally are low in fiber, move out of the stomach quickly, leaving you hungry.

But the process is more complicated than this. It has been found that high-GI meals actually trigger a series of hormonal and metabolic changes that promote overeating. In one study, subjects were broken into groups, with one group receiving a meal of low-GI foods, and another group, a meal of high-GI foods. After the meal, as expected, levels of blood glucose and insulin were found to rise highest and fastest in those who had eaten high-GI foods. Then, within just a few hours, these levels dropped significantly, leading to a stress response indicated by a rise in adrenalin levels. The result? Later that day, when the subjects were allowed to eat any foods they wished, those who had eaten meals of high-GI foods consumed nearly *twice as much* as those who had eaten low-GI meals. Moreover, it has been found that the frequent consumption of high-GI meals can result in perpetually high levels of insulin, perpetual hunger, and—as a result—frequent overeating.

Finally, it should be noted that when blood sugar levels rise, insulin brings blood sugar down primarily by converting the excess sugar to stored fat. This, clearly, can contribute to excess weight.

How are high-GI foods associated with cardiovascular disease?

Cardiovascular disease is the number-one cause of death in the United States. And there is growing evidence that diet and lifestyle are the causes of most cardiovascular disease. While most people know about the connection between heart disease and excess fat consumption, it's important to understand that diets high in fat often also provide large amounts of high-GI foods, such as refined wheat breads, white potatoes, and sugary soft drinks and desserts. Beyond that, The Nurses' Health Study found a clear link between a diet of high-GI foods and heart disease. Specifically, the study found that women with the highest dietary glycemic load (GL) have double the risk of heart disease compared with those with the lowest dietary glycemic load. (To learn about glycemic load, see page 17.) In fact, high-GL diets—and, therefore, diets composed mostly of high-GI foods—were found to be associated with lower concentrations of high-density lipoproteins (the so-called "good" cholesterol) as well as higher levels of triglycerides (markers of coronary artery disease). Similar results were found in the EURODIAB study, which looked at over 3,000 individuals from sixteen European countries. This study confirmed that higher levels of healthy high-density lipoproteins are found in people who consume diets rich in low-glycemic index foods.

It is also important to note that obesity is an important determinant of cardiovascular disease. The risk estimates of hypertension (high blood pressure), for instance, suggest that about 75 percent of hypertension can be attributed to obesity. Increased weight is also a determinant of higher levels of triglycerides, lower levels of high-density lipoproteins, and elevated levels of low-density lipoproteins (the "bad" cholesterol). Since we know that a diet of high-GI foods contributes to obesity, the link between high-GI foods and cardiovascular disorders is even easier to understand.

How are high-GI foods associated with metabolic syndrome?

Now that you have learned a little about the association between high-GI foods and the risk of diabetes, obesity, and cardiovascular disease, it makes sense to turn our attention to a condition known as *metabolic syndrome* or *syndrome X*. While you may have never heard about this condition, it is one that is attracting growing attention in the world of health.

Metabolic syndrome is actually a cluster of symptoms that include insulin resistance, high blood pressure, high cholesterol, high triglycerides, and increased weight. People with metabolic syndrome have been found to be at increased risk of coronary heart disease, stroke, and diabetes. It is estimated that 20 to 25 percent of adults in the United States have this syndrome.

Researchers have found that metabolic syndrome is closely related to insulin resistance—the condition discussed earlier, in which the body cannot use insulin efficiently. While some people are genetically predisposed to insulin resistance, as you know, much of the blame for this condition can be placed on the excessive consumption of high-GI foods. In fact, some experts have called metabolic syndrome a disease of overconsumption—overconsumption of high-glycemic index carbohydrates.

How are high-GI foods associated with cancer?

Several studies have shown a strong link between high-glycemic index foods and the incidence of colon cancer. In fact, researchers at Harvard and UCLA have found that the risk of colorectal cancer is nearly three times higher in women whose diets contain a high proportion of high glycemic-load foods compared with those who eat lesser amounts. In some women, the risk is six times higher.

Researchers have learned that this connection is caused by the tendency of high-GI foods to trigger insulin resistance. Insulin resistance, in turn, creates an environment in the colon that is conducive to tumor growth. And scientists don't believe that colon cancer is the only cancer associated with a high-GI diet. There is also evidence that high-GI foods boost the risk of both pancreatic cancer and breast cancer.

How are high-GI foods associated with fatigue?

Unlike diabetes, heart disease, and cancer, fatigue is not life-threatening. Yet it does impair quality of life for many people. And frequently, fatigue is the direct result of a diet that contains too many high-GI foods.

As you've learned, when a high-glycemic index food is consumed, it is quickly metabolized, resulting in a pronounced spike in blood sugar. While this rise in blood sugar causes an increase in energy, it is quickly followed by a spike in insulin production, which causes blood sugar levels to drop below normal, resulting in fatigue. Frequently, a vicious cycle is created in which an individual eats a high-GI food such as donuts for an energy boost, feels tired again when his or her blood sugar drops, reaches for another sweet in an effort to fight fatigue . . . and on and on.

How can a low-GI diet improve your health?

On the whole, your body performs best when your blood sugar is kept as constant as possible. When blood sugar drops too low, you become lethargic and may experience increased hunger. When blood sugar rises too high, the brain signals the pancreas to secrete more insulin, which, as you've learned, can lead to a number of problems. This is true both for healthy people and for people who are coping with various health disorders, which means that a diet of low-GI foods makes sense for everyone. In fact, it even makes sense for cats and dogs, who *must* eat a low-GI diet to maintain good health. When they don't, excess weight, diabetes, heart disease, and even cancer can result—just as they can in humans.

Earlier, you learned that the glycemic index was originally invented to help diabetes patients manage their blood sugar levels, and by now it should be clear that a diet which includes primarily low-GI foods benefits the diabetic patient by releasing energy slowly and steadily, and preventing spikes of blood glucose. Studies have demonstrated that lower-glycemic index foods both help control type II diabetes and reduce the symptoms of insulin resistance.

But a diet of lower-GI foods has been shown helpful in the management of other health problems, as well. For instance, low-GI foods have been found to help prevent coronary heart disease in both people with diabetes and healthy individuals. And in the obese and overweight, low-GI foods increase the feeling of fullness and facilitate the moderation of food intake. One study, conducted by David S. Ludwig, illustrated both of these points. In this study, obese participants were broken into two groups. The first group was instructed to follow a traditional low-fat, low-calorie weight-loss diet. The second group, known as the slow-carb group, was instructed to eat nonstarchy vegetables, fruits, beans, nuts, and dairy products—slow-carb and no-carb foods. They were also instructed to eat carbs with protein and healthful fats at every meal and snack. And, unlike the first group, they were allowed to eat as much as they wanted. At the end of the year, the slow-carb group had lost slightly more weight than the reduced-calorie group. Just as significant, the slow-carb group had done better in terms of heart disease risk factors, showing a far more significant drop in triglycerides, for example. (The slow-carb group experienced a 37-percent drop, while the other group experienced only a 19-percent decrease.)

Low-GI foods are also a great prescription for people who suffer from fatigue. While high-GI foods provide a short burst of energy followed by fatigue and lethargy, foods that are low on the glycemic index often act as "time-release energy." As the food is slowly metabolized, the glucose is gradually released into the body, keeping energy levels even. The truth is that glucose isn't bad—we need it to produce energy for every cell in our body. What we don't need is a rapid rise in blood sugar, followed by a spike in insulin.

Before we leave the subject of health disorders and the glycemic index, it makes sense to point out that many low-glycemic index foods are just plain healthier for us than higher-glycemic index foods. Just think about fresh fruits and vegetables, as well as beans, nuts, and whole grains—foods that, for the most part, are low-GI selections when eaten in their natural (unprocessed) state. These are the foods that provide us with an abundance of fiber, vitamins, and minerals, as well as beneficial compounds such as phytochemicals and antioxidants. These are also the foods that contribute to healthy body weight by preventing the storage of fat that's triggered by high-GI foods. As soon as we start adulterating these foods by refining the grains or cooking the fruits with sugar, for instance, they simultaneously rise higher on the index and become generally less healthy for us, as essential nutrients are stripped away and unhealthy ingredients are added to the mix. For this reason, it just makes sense to select low-glycemic index foods whenever possible. In fact, research has shown that we were genetically programmed to eat and thrive on a low-GI diet.

But it should also be noted that when eating for good health, the glycemic index is not the only factor that should be kept in mind. Some critics have pointed out that if you look solely at the GI when choosing your diet, you can easily end up overconsuming fats and total calories. You might even include an insufficient amount of important nutrients like carotenoids in your diet. That's why it's important to recognize that the glycemic index is just one tool, although a powerful one, when making food selections. It's vital to look at the total picture when choosing your diet, and to make sure that you're getting all the essential nutrients without eating too much of one type of food or consuming an excessive number of calories.

PART TWO

THE
GLYCEMIC INDEX
FOOD GUIDE

HOW TO USE
THIS TABLE

The table that begins on page 37 provides the glycemic index for a wide range of common foods and beverages. In addition to including whole uncooked foods, such as apples, it also lists some popular cooked, combination, and prepared foods, such as stir-fried vegetables with chicken. Foods are listed alphabetically under their name, and for ease of use, are also listed under their relevant categories. For instance, "Banana" can be found under both "Banana" and "Fruit," and "Udon noodles" can be found under "Udon," "Noodles," and "Asian Foods."

For each of the foods included, the table first provides the portion size and then tells you whether the food is Low GI (between 0 and 55), Mid-GI (56 to 69), or High GI (70 to 100) on the glycemic scale. The table uses these ratings, rather than a number, because of the variations you're likely to find in most foods due to factors such as the area in which the food was grown. Because such variations can have a significant effect on the carbohydrate content of the food and, therefore, the impact it has on glucose levels, the Low, Mid-, and High ratings provide a more realistic assessment of the food's glycemic index. For similar reasons, sometimes two boxes, such as Low GI and Mid-GI, are marked for a single food. This signifies that the food's impact on blood glucose levels can actually range from low to medium.

In some cases, a food is marked Insignificant Carbs rather than Low, Mid-, or High. This indicates that the food provides either no carbohydrates or such an insignificant amount of carbohydrates that it is believed to have no impact on blood sugar levels. Beef, for instance, falls into this category. (See pages 14 and 15 for more information on these foods.)

The last column in the table shows the food's glycemic load (GL). As explained on page 17, this gives you a fuller picture of that food than you would get from the glycemic index alone, by telling you how much of that carbohydrate is found in the serving size indicated. A GL of 10 or less is considered low, a GL of 11 to 19 is moderate, and one of 20 or more is high.

Once you have found a food in the table and learned its glycemic index, keep in mind that while the glycemic index is a wonderful tool, it has its limitations. As you've already learned, a single food's GI can vary widely depending on a number of factors, such as where it was grown and how it was prepared. Moreover, unless you eat that food entirely on its own, without consuming any other foods at the same time, its GI will be changed. Generally, the addition of fiber, protein, or fat reduces the GI of a food. Healthy eating is, to a degree, a balancing act. You can healthfully offset the high GI of one food by pairing it with a second food (or foods) that contributes GI-lowering fiber to the mix. You can also minimize the impact of a high-GI food by limiting portion size.

Finally, as discussed on page 30, you should not rely solely on GI or GL to choose your foods, as doing so can lead to an excessive consumption of fats and calories, and even the avoidance of certain nutrient-rich foods. By all means, use the glycemic index as an important guide, but make sure you eat a balanced diet that provides healthful portions of all essential nutrients.

GLYCEMIC INDEX

Food	Portion Size	Low GI (0–55)	Mid-GI (56–69)	High GI (70–100)	GL
Alcoholic beverages, all types	Standard	Insignificant Carbs			—

FAQ	Why don't alcoholic beverages have GI numbers? Aren't they made from high-carbohydrate ingredients? (See page 15.)

Food	Portion Size	Low GI (0–55)	Mid-GI (56–69)	High GI (70–100)	GL
Ale	Standard	Insignificant Carbs			—
All-Bran cereal (Kellogg's)					
Bran Buds	1 oz		▓		7
Bran Buds with psyllium	1 oz	▓			6
Bran Flakes	1 oz			▓	13
original	1 oz	▓			9
Almonds	Standard	Insignificant Carbs			—
Alpen Muesli cereal (Weetabix)	1 oz	▓			10
Amaranth chapatti bread	2 oz	▓			20
Angel food cake	1¾ oz		▓		19
Apple cinnamon snack bar (Con Agra)	1⅔ oz	▓			12
Apple muffins					
with sugar	2 oz / 1 muffin		▓		13
without sugar	2 oz / 1 muffin	▓			9
Apple juice, unsweetened	8¾ oz	▓			12
Apples					

Food	Portion Size	Low GI (0–55)	Mid-GI (56–69)	High GI (70–100)	GL
dried	²/₃ oz	■			5
fresh	4¹/₅ oz	■			6
Apricots					
canned in light syrup	4¹/₅ oz		■		12
dried	2 oz	■			9
fresh	4¹/₅ oz		■		5
Arborio rice, boiled (risotto)	5¹/₄ oz		■		36
Arrowroot cookies (McCormicks)	1 oz		■		13
Arrowroot plus cookies (McCormicks)	1 oz			■	11
Artichokes	Standard	Insignificant Carbs			—

ARTIFICIAL SWEETENERS (*See also* Sweeteners)					
Aspartame (NutraSweet)	Standard	Insignificant Carbs			—
Sucralose (Splenda)	Standard	Insignificant Carbs			—

Arugula	Standard	Insignificant Carbs			—

ASIAN FOODS					
Beans					
lentils, green	5¹/₄ oz	■			5

Food	Portion Size	Low GI (0–55)	Mid-GI (56–69)	High GI (70–100)	GL
lentils, red	5¼ oz	■			5
mung, boiled	5¼ oz	■			5
mung, sprouted	5¼ oz	■			4
Bok choy	Standard	Insignificant Carbs			—
Crackers, rice (sembei)	1 oz			■	23
Daikon radish	Standard	Insignificant Carbs			—
Lychees, canned in syrup and drained	4⅕ oz			■	16
Noodles					
brown rice	6⅓ oz			■	35
mung bean	6⅓ oz	■			14
udon, plain	6⅓ oz	■			23
vermicelli, durum wheat	5 oz	■			15
vermicelli, white	6⅓ oz	■			16
white rice	6⅓ oz		■		23
Rice					
broken, white, and cooked in rice cooker	5¼ oz			■	37
curry	5¼ oz		■		41
curry, with cheese	5¼ oz		■		27
jasmine, cooked in rice cooker	5¼ oz			■	46
sticky	5¼ oz			■	44

Food	Portion Size	Low GI (0–55)	Mid-GI (56–69)	High GI (70–100)	GL
white, with butter	5¼ oz			▓	40
Rice balls, Japanese (mochi)					
plain	2½ oz	▓			14
plain roasted	2½ oz			▓	21
salted and roasted	2½ oz			▓	20
Soup with soba noodles, instant	6⅓ oz	▓			22
Sprouts, mung bean	5¼ oz	▓			4
Sushi					
salmon	3½ oz	▓			17
sea algae, roasted with vinegar and rice	3½ oz	▓			20
Vegetables, stir-fried, with chicken and rice	12½ oz		▓		55
Aspartame (NutraSweet) (*See also* Sweeteners)	Standard	Insignificant Carbs			—
Avocados	Standard	Insignificant Carbs			—
Bagels, frozen white (Lender's)	2½ oz			▓	25
Baguette, plain white	1 oz			▓	15
Baked beans, canned					
haricot, in tomato sauce	5¼ oz	▓			7
navy, in tomato sauce	5¼ oz	▓			7

Baked goods (*See* Bagels; Biscuits; Breads; Cakes; Crackers; Crisp Breads; Donuts; Muffins; Rolls)

Food	Portion Size	Low GI (0–55)	Mid-GI (56–69)	High GI (70–100)	GL
Banana bread (cake)					
with sugar	2⁴/₅ oz	▓			18
without sugar	2⁴/₅ oz	▓			16
Banana smoothie, soy	8³/₄ oz	▓			7
Bananas					
over-ripe (yellow with brown)	4¹/₅ oz	▓			13
ripe (yellow)	4¹/₅ oz	▓			11
under-ripe (yellow with green)	4¹/₅ oz	▓			11
Barley	5¹/₄ oz	▓			26
Barley, pearl	5¹/₄ oz	▓			11
Barley chapatti bread	2 oz	▓			20
Barley flour	1 oz			▓	14
Basmati rice, white					
boiled	5¹/₄ oz	▓			22
microwaved in pouch (Uncle Ben's)	5¹/₄ oz	▓			24
quick-cooking, cooked 10 minutes (Uncle Ben's)	5¹/₄ oz		▓		23
Batavia endive (escarole)	Standard	Insignificant Carbs			—

BEANS AND LEGUMES

Baked, canned

Food	Portion Size	Low GI (0–55)	Mid-GI (56–69)	High GI (70–100)	GL
haricot beans, in tomato sauce	5¼ oz	■			7
navy beans, in tomato sauce	5¼ oz	■			7
Boiled					
black beans	5¼ oz	■			7
black-eyed peas (cowpeas)	5¼ oz	■			13
broad beans	2⅘ oz		■		9
brown beans	5¼ oz	■			9
cannellini beans, canned	3 oz	■			5
chickpeas (garbanzo), in brine	5¼ oz	■			9
chickpeas (garbanzo), in curry	5¼ oz	■			7
chickpeas (garbanzo), plain	5¼ oz	■			9
green peas, frozen	2⅘ oz	■			3
haricot beans	5¼ oz	■			9
kidney beans	5¼ oz	■			7
lentils, green	5¼ oz	■			5
lentils, red	5¼ oz	■			5
lima beans (butter beans)	5¼ oz	■			6
lima beans (butter beans), sugar added	5¼ oz	■			6
marrowfat peas	5¼ oz	■			7
mung beans	5¼ oz	■			5

Food	Portion Size	Low GI (0–55)	Mid-GI (56–69)	High GI (70–100)	GL
navy beans	5¼ oz				9
pinto beans, in brine	5¼ oz				4
pinto beans, plain	5¼ oz				10
romano beans	4 oz				8
snap peas	4 oz / 1 cup				10
soy beans	5¼ oz				1
split peas	4 oz				6
Pressure-cooked					
haricot beans	5¼ oz				12
mung beans	5¼ oz				7
navy beans	5¼ oz				12
Sprouted					
mung beans	5¼ oz				4

FAQ	Why isn't beef ranked on the GI? (See page 14.)

BEEF			
Bologna, 100% meat	Standard	Insignificant Carbs	—
Frankfurter, 100% meat	Standard	Insignificant Carbs	—
Hamburger, 100% meat	Standard	Insignificant Carbs	—

Food	Portion Size	Low GI (0–55)	Mid-GI (56–69)	High GI (70–100)	GL
Liver	Standard	Insignificant Carbs			—
Steak	Standard	Insignificant Carbs			—

FAQ	Since beer contains an insignificant amount of carbs, can I drink as much as I want? (See pages 15 and 16.)

Food	Portion Size	Low GI (0–55)	Mid-GI (56–69)	High GI (70–100)	GL
Beer	Standard	Insignificant Carbs			—
Beetroot (*See* Beets)					
Beets	2⁴/₅ oz		5		5
Belgian endive (witloof)	Standard	Insignificant Carbs			—

BERRIES					
Blueberries	8 oz		5		5
Raspberries	8 oz	5			5
Strawberries	4¹/₅ oz	1			1

BEVERAGES					
Ale	Standard	Insignificant Carbs			—
Apple juice, unsweetened	8³/₄ oz	12			12
Beer	Standard	Insignificant Carbs			—
Blueberry juice	8³/₄ oz		14		14

Food	Portion Size	Low GI (0–55)	Mid-GI (56–69)	High GI (70–100)	GL
Carrot juice, fresh and unsweetened	8¾ oz	■			10
Chocolate Quik					
made with 1.5%-fat milk	8¾ oz	■			5
made with water	8¾ oz	■			4
Cola (Coca-Cola)					
Diet Coke	Standard	Insignificant Carbs			—
regular Coke	12 oz		■		16
Cranberry Juice Cocktail (Ocean Spray)	8¾ oz			■	24
Gatorade	8¾ oz			■	12
Grape juice	8¾ oz		■		24
Grapefruit juice	8¾ oz	■			11
Hot chocolate, made with water (Nestlé)	8¾ oz	■			11
Lemonade	6 oz		■		13
Liquor, all varieties	Standard	Insignificant Carbs			—
Malt liquor	Standard	Insignificant Carbs			—
Milk					
buttermilk	8¾ oz	■			5
chocolate	1¾ oz	■			12
condensed, sweetened (Nestlé)	1¾ oz		■		17
skim	8¾ oz	■			4

Food	Portion Size	Low GI (0–55)	Mid-GI (56–69)	High GI (70–100)	GL
soy, full-fat	8¾ oz	■			8
soy, reduced-fat	8¾ oz	■			8
whole	8¾ oz	■			3
Orange juice					
fresh	8¾ oz	■			12
from frozen concentrate	8¾ oz		■		15
unsweetened, reconstituted	8¾ oz	■			9
Orange soda (Fanta)	8¾ oz			■	23
Pineapple juice, unsweetened (Dole)	8¾ oz	■			16
Pomegranate juice	8¾ oz		■		23
Seltzer	Standard	Insignificant Carbs			—
Smoothie drinks					
banana, soy	8¾ oz	■			7
raspberry (Con Agra)	8¾ oz	■			14
Strawberry Quik					
made with 1.5%-fat milk	8¾ oz	■			4
made with water	8¾ oz		■		5
Tea	Standard	Insignificant Carbs			—
Tomato juice, unsweetened	8¾ oz	■			4
Tonic water (Schweppes)	8¾ oz		■		17
Wine	Standard	Insignificant Carbs			—

Food	Portion Size	Low GI (0–55)	Mid-GI (56–69)	High GI (70–100)	GL
BISCUITS (*See also* Breads)					
Croissants	2 oz		■		17
Crumpets	1¾ oz		■		13
Scones, plain from premix	1 oz			■	8
Black bean soup	8¾ oz		■		17
Black beans, boiled	5¼ oz	■			7
Black-eyed peas, boiled	5¼ oz	■			13
Blueberries	8 oz		■		5
Blueberry juice	8¾ oz		■		14
Blueberry muffins	2 oz / 1 muffin		■		17
Bok choy	Standard	Insignificant Carbs			—
Bologna, 100% meat	Standard	Insignificant Carbs			—
Bourbon (liquor)	Standard	Insignificant Carbs			—
Bran Buds cereal, All-Bran (Kellogg's)	1 oz		■		7
Bran Buds cereal with psyllium, All-Bran (Kellogg's)	1 oz	■			6
Bran Chex cereal (Nabisco)	1 oz		■		11
Bran Flakes cereal, All-Bran (Kellogg's)	1 oz			■	13
Bran muffins	2 oz / 1 muffin		■		15

Food	Portion Size	Low GI (0–55)	Mid-GI (56–69)	High GI (70–100)	GL
Breadfruit	4⅕ oz		▓		18

TIP	When buying bread, look for a whole grain variety that has been processed as little as possible and has 3 to 4 grams of fiber per slice. Cracked or sprouted whole wheat breads are often a good low-GI choice. (For more information, see page 19.)

BREADS (*See also* Biscuits; Crisp Breads; Rolls)					
Bagel, frozen white (Lender's)	2½ oz			▓	25
Baguette, plain white	1 oz			▓	15
Banana bread					
with sugar	2⅘ oz	▓			18
without sugar	2⅘ oz	▓			16
Buckwheat	1 oz / 1 slice	▓			10
Bulgur	1 oz / 1 slice	▓			11
Chapatti (Indian bread)					
amaranth	2 oz		▓		20
barley	2 oz	▓			20
wheat	2 oz			▓	21
English muffin	1 oz / 1 muffin			▓	11
Healthy Choice (Con Agra)					

Food	Portion Size	Low GI (0–55)	Mid-GI (56–69)	High GI (70–100)	GL
Hearty 100% Whole Grain	1 oz / 1 slice		■		9
Hearty 7 Grain	1 oz / 1 slice	■			8
Lebanese bread	1 oz			■	12
Linseed rye, whole grain	1 oz / 1 slice	■			7
Multigrain bread					
9-grain	1 oz / 1 slice	■			6
gluten-free	1 oz / 1 slice			■	10
Oat bran	1 oz / 1 slice	■			6
Pita bread					
wheat	1 oz		■		10
white	1 oz		■		10
Pumpernickel, whole grain	1 oz / 1 slice	■			5
Raisin bread	1 oz / 1 slice		■		10
Rye					
cocktail	1 oz / 1 slice	■			7
kernel	1 oz / 1 slice	■			5
light	1 oz / 1 slice		■		10
linseed, whole grain	1 oz / 1 slice	■			8
sourdough	1 oz / 1 slice		■		6
whole grain	1 oz / 1 slice		■		8
Sourdough					

Food	Portion Size	Low GI (0–55)	Mid-GI (56–69)	High GI (70–100)	GL
rye	1 oz / 1 slice	▓			6
wheat	1 oz / 1 slice	▓			6
Soy and linseed	1 oz / 1 slice	▓			6
Spelt					
multigrain	1 oz / 1 slice	▓			7
white	1 oz / 1 slice	▓			17
whole grain	1 oz / 1 slice		▓		12
Turkish					
white-wheat	1 oz / 1 slice			▓	15
whole wheat	1 oz / 1 slice	▓			8
Wheat					
coarse kernel	1 oz / 1 slice	▓			10
sourdough	1 oz / 1 slice	▓			6
whole wheat, 100%	1 oz / 1 slice			▓	10
White					
gluten-free	1 oz / 1 slice			▓	11
regular (Wonder)	1 oz / 1 slice			▓	10
whole wheat	1 oz / 1 slice		▓		10
Whole grain, 100%	1 oz / 1 slice	▓			5

Breakfast foods (*See* Breads; Cereals; Crisp Breads; Fruit)

Food	Portion Size	Low GI (0–55)	Mid-GI (56–69)	High GI (70–100)	GL
Breton wheat crackers (Dare)	1 oz		▓		10
Broad beans, boiled	2⁴/₅ oz		▓	▓	9
Broccoli	Standard	Insignificant Carbs			—
Broccoli rabe (rapini)	Standard	Insignificant Carbs			—
Brown beans, boiled	5¼ oz	▓			9
Brown rice					
boiled	5¼ oz		▓		21
parboiled and cooked 20 min	5¼ oz		▓		23
steamed	5¼ oz	▓			16
Brussels sprouts	Standard	Insignificant Carbs			—
Buckwheat	5¼ oz		▓		16
Buckwheat bread	1 oz / 1 slice		▓		10
Bulgur bread	1 oz / 1 slice		▓		11
Bulgur wheat, boiled	1¾ oz	▓			12
Burger (*See* Hamburger patty)					
Butter	Standard	Insignificant Carbs			—
Butter beans, boiled (lima beans)					
with no added sugar	5¼ oz	▓			6
with sugar added	5¼ oz	▓			6
Buttermilk	8¾ oz	▓			5
Cabbage	Standard	Insignificant Carbs			—

Food	Portion Size	Low GI (0–55)	Mid-GI (56–69)	High GI (70–100)	GL
Cactus pear (nopal)	Standard	Insignificant Carbs			—

CAKES (*See also* Desserts)					
Angel food cake	1¾ oz		▓		19
Banana bread (cake)					
with sugar	3 oz	▓			18
without sugar	3 oz	▓			16
Chocolate cake with frosting	4 oz	▓			20
Flan cake	2½ oz		▓		31
Pound cake	2 oz	▓			15
Sponge cake	2⅕ oz	▓			17
Vanilla cake with frosting	4 oz	▓			24

Cajun Style rice (Uncle Ben's)	5¼ oz	▓			19

CANDY (*See also* Energy bars; Fruit bars; Snack bars)					
Candy bars					
Mars (Mars)	2 oz		▓	▓	27
Snickers (Mars)	2 oz		▓		23
Twix (Mars)	2 oz	▓			17
Jelly beans	1 oz			▓	22

Food	Portion Size	Low GI (0–55)	Mid-GI (56–69)	High GI (70–100)	GL
Life Savers (Nestlé)	1 oz		▓		21
M&M's, Peanut (Mars)	1 oz	▓			6
Marshmallows	1			▓	5
Skittles (Mars)	1 2/3 oz		▓		32

Cannellini beans, boiled	3 oz	▓			5
Cantaloupe	4 1/5 oz		▓		4
Capellini pasta	6 1/3 oz	▓			20
Carob	1/4 oz	▓			5
Carrot juice, fresh and unsweetened	8 3/4 oz	▓			10
Carrot muffins	2 oz / 1 muffin		▓		20

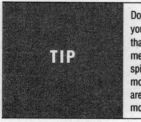

TIP

Don't let the carrot's high-GI rating discourage you from eating this nutritious food. Note that carrots have a low glycemic. This means that you have to eat a lot to cause a spike in blood sugar levels. When eaten in moderation as part of a low-GI diet, carrots are a valuable addition to your diet. (For more information, see page 18.)

Carrots					
cooked	2 2/3 oz		▓		5
fresh	2 4/5 oz			▓	5

Food	Portion Size	Low GI (0–55)	Mid-GI (56–69)	High GI (70–100)	GL
Cashews, salted	1³/₄ oz	■			3
Cassava, boiled	2⁴/₅ oz	■			12
Cauliflower	Standard	Insignificant Carbs			—
Celery	Standard	Insignificant Carbs			—

CEREAL (*See also* Grains)					
All-Bran (Kellogg's)					
Bran Buds	1 oz		■		7
Bran Buds with psyllium	1 oz	■			6
Bran Flakes	1 oz			■	13
original	1 oz	■			9
Bran Chex (Nabisco)	1 oz		■		11
Cheerios (General Mills)	1 oz			■	15
Coco Pops (Kellogg's)	1 oz			■	20
Corn Bran (Quaker Oats)	1 oz			■	15
Corn Chex (Nabisco)	1 oz			■	21
Corn Flakes (Kellogg's)	1 oz			■	24
Cream of Wheat (Nabisco)					
instant	8³/₄ oz			■	22
regular	8³/₄ oz		■		17
Crispix (Kellogg's)	1 oz			■	22

Food	Portion Size	Low GI (0–55)	Mid-GI (56–69)	High GI (70–100)	GL
Froot Loops (Kellogg's)	1 oz		■		18
Frosties (Kellogg's)	1 oz	■			15
Golden Grahams (General Mills)	1 oz			■	18
Grape-Nuts (Post)	1 oz			■	15
Grape-Nuts Flakes (Post)	1 oz			■	17
Life (Quaker Oats)	1 oz		■		16
Mini-Wheats (Kellogg's)	4 oz		■		10
Muesli, Alpen (Weetabix)	1 oz	■			10
Oat Bran (Quaker)	⅓ oz	■			2
Oatmeal, instant (Quaker)	8¾ oz		■		17
Oatmeal, regular					
barley	1¾ oz		■		17
rolled oats	8¾ oz		■		17
Puffed Wheat (Quaker)	1 oz		■		13
Raisin Bran (Kellogg's)	1 oz		■		12
Red River Cereal (Maple Leaf Mills)	1 oz	■			11
Rice Chex (Nabisco)	1 oz			■	23
Rice Krispies (Kellogg's)	1 oz			■	21
Shredded Wheat (Nabisco)	1 oz			■	15
Special K (Kellogg's)	1 oz		■		14
Team Flakes (Nabisco)	1 oz			■	17

Food	Portion Size	Low GI (0–55)	Mid-GI (56–69)	High GI (70–100)	GL
Total (General Mills)	1 oz			▓	17
Weetabix (Weetabix)	1 oz		▓		16
Cereal bars (*See* Energy bars; Fruit bars; Snack bars)					
Chapatti (Indian bread)					
amaranth	2 oz			▓	20
barley	2 oz	▓			20
wheat	2 oz	▓			21
Chard, Swiss	Standard	Insignificant Carbs			—
Cheerios cereal (General Mills)	1 oz			▓	15
Cheese	Standard	Insignificant Carbs			—
Cheese pizza					
regular crust	3½ oz		▓		16
with tomato sauce, regular crust	3½ oz			▓	22
with tomato sauce, thin crust	3½ oz	▓			7
with tomato sauce, vegetables, thin crust	3½ oz	▓			12
Cheese tortellini	6⅓ oz	▓			10
Cherries, fresh	4⅕ oz	▓			3
CHICKEN					
Liver	Standard	Insignificant Carbs			—

Food	Portion Size	Low GI (0–55)	Mid-GI (56–69)	High GI (70–100)	GL
Nuggets, microwavable	3½ oz	▓			7
Parts	Standard	Insignificant Carbs			—
Roll, 100% meat	Standard	Insignificant Carbs			—

Chickpeas, boiled (garbanzo beans)

in brine	5¼ oz	▓			9
in curry	5¼ oz	▓			7
plain	5¼ oz	▓			9

TIP

Like other leafy greens, chicory is a neutral food, meaning that it contains little or no carbs and is not likely to have an effect on your blood sugar level. Chicory is also a healthy food that can be enjoyed all day long.

Chicory	Standard	Insignificant Carbs			—
Chicory, red leaf (radicchio)	Standard	Insignificant Carbs			—

Chinese foods (*See* Asian Foods)

Chinese radish	Standard	Insignificant Carbs			—

Chips

corn, salted	1¾ oz		▓		17
potato, plain salted	1¾ oz	▓			11
tortilla	1¾ oz		▓		17

Food	Portion Size	Low GI (0–55)	Mid-GI (56–69)	High GI (70–100)	GL
Chocolate cake with frosting	4 oz	■			20
Chocolate candy					
M&M's, Peanut (Mars)	1 oz	■			6
Mars bar (Mars)	2 oz		■		27
Snickers bar (Mars)	2 oz			■	23
Twix (Mars)	2 oz	■			17
CHOCOLATE DRINKS					
Chocolate milk	1¾ oz	■			12
Chocolate Quik (Nestlé)					
made with 1.5%-fat milk	8¾ oz	■			5
made with water	8¾ oz	■			4
Dutch Chocolate (Usana)	8¾ oz	■			4
Hot chocolate, made with water (Nestlé)	8¾ oz	■			11
Chocolate ice cream					
high-fat (premium, 15% fat)	1¾ oz	■			4
reduced-fat (1.4% fat)	1¾ oz	■			5
regular-fat	1¾ oz		■		8
Chocolate pudding, from premix	4 oz	■			10
Chocolate substitute (*See* Carob)					

Food	Portion Size	Low GI (0–55)	Mid-GI (56–69)	High GI (70–100)	GL
Choice nutritional drink (Mead Johnson)	7 oz	▨			6

CITRUS FRUITS					
Grapefruit	4⅕ oz	▨			3
Orange	4⅕ oz	▨			5

Clams	Standard	Insignificant Carbs			—
Coca-Cola (*See* Cola; Soft Drinks)					
Coco Pops cereal (Kellogg's)	1 oz			▨	20
Coke (*See* Cola; Soft Drinks)					
Cola (Coca-Cola)					
Diet Coke	Standard	Insignificant Carbs			—
regular Coke	12 oz		▨		16

COLD CUTS, 100% MEAT					
Bologna	Standard	Insignificant Carbs			—
Chicken	Standard	Insignificant Carbs			—
Ham	Standard	Insignificant Carbs			—
Liverwurst	Standard	Insignificant Carbs			—
Pastrami	Standard	Insignificant Carbs			—
Salami	Standard	Insignificant Carbs			—

Food	Portion Size	Low GI (0–55)	Mid-GI (56–69)	High GI (70–100)	GL
Turkey	Standard	Insignificant Carbs			—
Collard greens	Standard	Insignificant Carbs			—
Condensed milk, sweetened (Nestlé)	1¾ oz		■		17

CONDIMENTS					
Mayonnaise					
Hellman's	Standard	Insignificant Carbs			—
Weight Watchers	Standard	Insignificant Carbs			—
Mustard	Standard	Insignificant Carbs			—
Pepper, black	Standard	Insignificant Carbs			—
Salt	Standard	Insignificant Carbs			—

COOKIES (*See also* Desserts)					
Arrowroot (McCormicks)	1 oz		■		13
Arrowroot plus (McCormicks)	1 oz		■		11
Graham Wafers (Christie Brown & Co.)	1 oz			■	14
Oatmeal	1 oz	■			9
Peek Freans (Nabisco)	1 oz		■		10
Rich Tea	1 oz	■			10

Food	Portion Size	Low GI (0–55)	Mid-GI (56–69)	High GI (70–100)	GL
Vanilla Wafers (Christie Brown & Co.)	1 oz			■	14
Corn, sweet					
canned, diet pack	2⁴/₅ oz	■			7
frozen, microwavable	2⁴/₅ oz	■			7
on cob, boiled 20 minutes	2⁴/₅ oz		■		11
Corn Bran cereal (Quaker Oats)	1 oz			■	15
Corn Chex cereal (Nabisco)	1 oz			■	21
Corn chips, salted	1³/₄ oz		■		17
Corn Flakes cereal (Kellogg's)	1 oz			■	24
Corn muffins, with low amylose	2 oz / 1 muffin			■	30
Corn pasta, gluten-free	6¹/₃ oz		■		32
Corn tortilla with refried pinto beans, tomato sauce	3¹/₂ oz	■			9
Corn tortilla, fried, with mashed potato, tomato, lettuce	3¹/₂ oz	■			11
Cornmeal	5¹/₄ oz			■	9
Couscous	5¹/₄ oz		■		23
Couscous, Moroccan, with semolina, chickpeas, veggies	8³/₄ oz		■		17
Cowpeas (*See* Black-eyed peas, boiled)					
Crabmeat	Standard	Insignificant Carbs			—

Food	Portion Size	Low GI (0–55)	Mid-GI (56–69)	High GI (70–100)	GL
FAQ	Does eating more of a food cause its GI ranking to rise higher? (See page 17.)				

CRACKERS (*See also* Crisp Breads)					
Breton wheat crackers (Dare)	1 oz		▒		10
Premium Soda Crackers (Christie Brown & Co.)	1 oz			▒	12
Rice crackers, plain (sembei)	1 oz			▒	23
Stoned Wheat Thins (Christie Brown & Co.)	1 oz		▒		12
Wheat Thins (Nabisco)	8 crackers		▒		7

Cranberry Juice Cocktail (Ocean Spray)	8¾ oz		▒		24
Cream, sour	Standard	Insignificant Carbs			—
Cream of Wheat cereal (Nabisco)					
instant	8¾ oz			▒	22
regular	8¾ oz			▒	17

CRISP BREADS (*See also* Crackers)					
Bran	1 oz / 1 biscuit	▒			5
Melba toast	1 oz			▒	16
Rye	1 oz		▒		11
Whole wheat snack (Ryvita)	1 oz			▒	16

Food	Portion Size	Low GI (0–55)	Mid-GI (56–69)	High GI (70–100)	GL
Crispix cereal (Kellogg's)	1 oz			■	22
Crisps, potato, plain salted	1¾ oz	■			11
Croissants	2 oz		■		17
Crumpets	1¾ oz		■		13
Cucumbers	Standard		Insignificant Carbs		—
Currants	½ oz		■		10
Curry rice	5¼ oz		■		41
Curry rice with cheese	5¼ oz	■			27
Custard, homemade with milk	3½ oz	■			7
Daikon radish	Standard		Insignificant Carbs		—
DAIRY PRODUCTS					
Cheese	Standard		Insignificant Carbs		—
Custard, homemade with milk	3½ oz	■			7
Ice cream					
high-fat chocolate (15% fat)	1¾ oz	■			4
high-fat French vanilla (16% fat)	1¾ oz	■			3
low-fat chocolate (1.4% fat)	1¾ oz	■			5
low-fat vanilla (1.2% fat)	1¾ oz	■			5
regular-fat chocolate	1¾ oz		■		8

Food	Portion Size	Low GI (0–55)	Mid-GI (56–69)	High GI (70–100)	GL
regular-fat half-vanilla, half-chocolate	1¾ oz		▓		8
regular-fat vanilla	1¾ oz		▓		8
Milk					
buttermilk	8¾ oz	▓			5
chocolate milk	1¾ oz	▓			12
condensed milk, sweetened (Nestlé)	1¾ oz		▓		17
fat-free milk	8¾ oz	▓			5
skim milk	8¾ oz	▓			4
whole milk	8¾ oz	▓			3
Sour cream	Standard	Insignificant Carbs			—
Tapioca pudding with milk	4½ oz			▓	40
Yogurt					
low-fat milk, plain, no sugar	6 oz	▓			5
low-fat milk, with artificial sweetener	7 oz	▓			2
low-fat milk, with sugar	7 oz	▓			10
non-fat milk, with artificial sweetener	7 oz	▓			3
reduced-fat milk, with fruit	7 oz	▓			7
whole milk, no sugar	7 oz	▓			3
Dandelion greens	Standard	Insignificant Carbs			—

Food	Portion Size	Low GI (0–55)	Mid-GI (56–69)	High GI (70–100)	GL
Dates, dried	2 oz			▓	42

DESSERTS					
Cakes					
angel food cake	1¾ oz		▓		19
banana bread with sugar	3 oz	▓			18
banana bread without sugar	3 oz	▓			16
chocolate cake with frosting	4 oz	▓			20
flan cake	2½ oz		▓		31
pound cake	2 oz	▓			15
sponge cake	2⅕ oz	▓			17
vanilla cake with frosting	4 oz	▓			24
Candy					
jelly beans	1 oz			▓	22
Life Savers (Nestlé)	1 oz			▓	21
M&M's, Peanut (Mars)	1 oz	▓			6
marshmallows	1			▓	5
Skittles (Mars)	1⅔ oz		▓		32
Candy bars					
Mars (Mars)	2 oz		▓		27
Snickers (Mars)	2 oz		▓		23

Food	Portion Size	Low GI (0–55)	Mid-GI (56–69)	High GI (70–100)	GL
Twix (Mars)	2 oz	■			17
Cookies					
Arrowroot (McCormicks)	1 oz		■		13
Arrowroot plus (McCormicks)	1 oz		■		11
Graham Wafers (Christie Brown & Co.)	1 oz			■	14
Oatmeal	1 oz	■			9
Peek Freans (Nabisco)	1 oz		■		10
Rich Tea	1 oz		■		10
Vanilla Wafers (Christie Brown & Co.)	1 oz			■	14
Donuts, plain cake	1⅔ oz			■	17
Ice cream					
high-fat chocolate (15% fat)	1¾ oz	■			4
high-fat French vanilla (16% fat)	1¾ oz	■			3
low-fat chocolate (1.4% fat)	1¾ oz	■			5
low-fat vanilla (1.2% fat)	1¾ oz	■			5
regular-fat chocolate	1¾ oz		■		8
regular-fat half-vanilla, half-chocolate	1¾ oz		■		8
regular-fat vanilla	1¾ oz		■		8
Muffins					
apple with sugar	2 oz / 1 muffin	■			13

Food	Portion Size	Low GI (0–55)	Mid-GI (56–69)	High GI (70–100)	GL
apple without sugar	2 oz / 1 muffin	■			9
blueberry	2 oz / 1 muffin		■		17
bran	2 oz / 1 muffin		■		15
carrot	2 oz / 1 muffin		■		20
corn, with low amylose	2 oz / 1 muffin			■	30
oatmeal	2 oz / 1 muffin	■			24
Puddings, custards, and mousse					
custard, homemade, with milk	3½ oz	■			7
mousse, instant reduced-fat, with water	1¾ oz	■			4
pudding, chocolate, from premix	4 oz	■			10
pudding, instant, with whole milk	3½ oz	■			7
pudding, vanilla, from premix	4 oz	■			9
Snack bars					
apple cinnamon (Con Agra)	1⅔ oz	■			12
peanut butter and chocolate chip (Con Agra)	1⅔ oz	■			10
Snack foods					
corn chips, salted	1¾ oz		■		17
Pop Tarts (Kellogg's)	1 pastry			■	25
popcorn, plain microwavable	1 oz			■	8
potato chips, plain salted	1¾ oz	■			11

Food	Portion Size	Low GI (0–55)	Mid-GI (56–69)	High GI (70–100)	GL
pretzels, wheat	1 oz			▓	16
tortilla chips	1¾ oz		▓		17
Tofu-based frozen dessert, chocolate	1¾ oz			▓	10

| **Diet Coke** (Coca-Cola) (*See also* Soft Drinks) | Standard | Insignificant Carbs | | | — |
| **Donuts, plain cake** | 1⅔ oz | | | ▓ | 17 |

Dressing, salad

| oil and vinegar | Standard | Insignificant Carbs | | | — |

DRIED FRUITS

Apples	⅔ oz	▓			20
Apricots	2 oz	▓			9
Dates	2 oz			▓	42
Figs	2 oz			▓	42
Prunes	4⅕ oz	▓			6
Raisins	2 oz		▓		28

Drink mixers (*See* Mixers, drink)

DRINKS MADE WITH POWDERED MIXES

Chocolate Quik (Nestlé)

Food	Portion Size	Low GI (0–55)	Mid-GI (56–69)	High GI (70–100)	GL
made with 1.5%-fat milk	8¾ oz	■			5
made with water	8¾ oz	■			4
Dutch Chocolate (Usana)	8¾ oz	■			4
Enercal Plus nutritional drink (Wyeth-Ayerst)	7 oz		■		24
Hot chocolate, made with water (Nestlé)	8¾ oz	■			11
Lemonade	6 oz		■		13
Strawberry Quik (Nestlé)					
made with 1.5%-fat milk	8¾ oz	■			4
made with water	8¾ oz	■			5
Duck	Standard	Insignificant Carbs			—
Egg noodles	2⅔ oz	■			5
Eggs	Standard	Insignificant Carbs			—
Endive, Batavia (*See* Escarole)					
Endive, Belgian (witloof)	Standard	Insignificant Carbs			—
Enercal Plus nutritional drink mix (Wyeth-Ayerst)	7 oz		■		24
Energy bars (*See also* Fruits bars; Snack bars)					
Ironman PR Bar, chocolate (PR Nutrition)	2¼ oz		■		10
Power Bar (Powerfood)	2¼ oz		■		24
English muffin	1 oz / 1 muffin			■	11

Food	Portion Size	Low GI (0–55)	Mid-GI (56–69)	High GI (70–100)	GL
Ensure nutritional drink (Abbott)	7 oz	■			19
Ensure Plus nutritional drink (Abbott)	4 oz	■			9
Escarole (Batavia endive)	Standard	Insignificant Carbs			—
Fettuccine, egg	6⅓ oz	■			15
Figs, dried	2 oz			■	42

FAQ	Why isn't fish ranked on the GI? (See page 14.)

FISH (*See also* Seafood)					
Fresh-water	Standard	Insignificant Carbs			—
Salt-water	Standard	Insignificant Carbs			—

Flan cake	2½ oz		■		31

Flapjacks (*See* Pancakes)

Flat bread (*See* Crisp Breads; Pita)

FLOUR					
Barley	1 oz			■	14
Soy	8 oz	■			10

Food	Portion Size	Low GI (0–55)	Mid-GI (56–69)	High GI (70–100)	GL
Frankfurter bun	1 bun		■		12
Frankfurters, 100% meat	Standard	Insignificant Carbs			—
French fries	5¼ oz			■	22
Froot Loops cereal (Kellogg's)	1 oz		■		18
Frosties cereal (Kellogg's)	1 oz	■			15
Frozen non-dairy dessert					
tofu-based, chocolate	1¾ oz			■	10
Fructose (*See also* Sweeteners)	⅓ oz	■			1

FRUIT (*See also* Fruit Juices)					
Apples					
dried	⅔ oz	■			20
fresh	4⅕ oz	■			6
Apricots					
canned in light syrup	4⅕ oz		■		12
dried	2 oz	■			9
fresh	4⅕ oz		■		5
Avocados	Standard	Insignificant Carbs			—
Bananas	4⅕ oz		■		12
Blueberries	8 oz	■			5
Breadfruit	4⅕ oz		■		18

Food	Portion Size	Low GI (0–55)	Mid-GI (56–69)	High GI (70–100)	GL
Cantaloupe	4⅕ oz		■		4
Cherries	4⅕ oz	■			3
Currants	½ oz		■		10
Dates, dried	2 oz			■	42
Grapefruit	4⅕ oz	■			3
Grapes					
dried (raisins)	2 oz		■		28
fresh	4⅕ oz	■			8
Honeydew	8 oz		■		5
Kiwi	4⅕ oz		■		6
Lychees, canned in syrup and drained	4⅕ oz			■	16
Mangos	4⅕ oz		■		8
Nopal (cactus pear)	Standard	Insignificant Carbs			—
Oranges	4⅕ oz	■			5
Papaya (paw paw)	4⅕ oz		■		10
Peaches					
canned in light syrup (Del Monte)	4⅕ oz		■		9
canned in natural juice	4⅕ oz	■			5
fresh	4⅕ oz	■			5
Pears					

Food	Portion Size	Low GI (0–55)	Mid-GI (56–69)	High GI (70–100)	GL
fresh	4$\frac{1}{5}$ oz	■			4
halves, canned in low-sugar syrup	4$\frac{1}{5}$ oz	■			4
halves, canned in natural juice	4$\frac{1}{5}$ oz	■			5
Pineapple					
canned in syrup	3 oz		■		15
fresh	4$\frac{1}{5}$ oz	■			7
Plums					
dried, pitted (prunes)	4$\frac{1}{5}$ oz	■			6
fresh	4$\frac{1}{5}$ oz	■			5
Prunes	4$\frac{1}{5}$ oz	■			6
Raisins	2 oz		■		28
Raspberries	8 oz	■			5
Strawberries	4$\frac{1}{5}$ oz	■			1
Watermelon	4$\frac{1}{5}$ oz			■	4
Fruit, dried (*See* Dried fruit)					
Fruit bars (*See also* Candy; Energy bars)					
apricot	1$\frac{3}{4}$ oz	■			17
strawberry	1 oz			■	23
Fruit cocktail (Del Monte)	4$\frac{1}{5}$ oz	■			9

Food	Portion Size	Low GI (0–55)	Mid-GI (56–69)	High GI (70–100)	GL
TIP	When buying fruit juices, buy unsweetened brands, as they are the lowest GI choices. As you might suspect, added sweeteners raise the GI.				

FRUIT JUICES					
Apple, unsweetened	8¾ oz	▓			12
Blueberry	8¾ oz		▓		14
Cranberry, cocktail (Ocean Spray)	8¾ oz		▓		24
Grape	8¾ oz		▓		24
Grapefruit, unsweetened	8¾ oz	▓			11
Orange					
fresh	8¾ oz	▓			12
frozen concentrate	8¾ oz		▓		15
unsweetened, reconstituted	8¾ oz	▓			9
Pineapple, unsweeteneed (Dole)	8¾ oz		▓		16
Pomegranate	8¾ oz		▓		23
Gatorade	8¾ oz			▓	12
Garbanzo beans, boiled (chickpeas)					
in brine	5¼ oz	▓			9
in curry	5¼ oz	▓			7

Food	Portion Size	Low GI (0–55)	Mid-GI (56–69)	High GI (70–100)	GL
plain	5¼ oz	▓			9
Garden Style rice (Uncle Ben's)	5¼ oz	▓			21
Gin (liquor)	Standard	Insignificant Carbs			—
Glucerna nutritional drink, vanilla (Abbott)	7 oz	▓			7
Glucose (*See also* Sweeteners)	⅓ oz			▓	10
Glutinous rice (sticky rice)	5¼ oz			▓	44
Gnocchi	6⅓ oz		▓		33
Golden Grahams cereal (General Mills)	1 oz			▓	18
Graham Wafers (Christie Brown & Co.)	1 oz			▓	14

GRAINS (*See also* Cereals; Rice)					
Barley	5¼ oz	▓			26
Barley, pearl	5¼ oz	▓			11
Buckwheat	5¼ oz	▓			16
Corn, sweet	5¼ oz		▓		20
Cornmeal	5¼ oz		▓		9
Couscous	5¼ oz		▓		23
Millet, boiled	5¼ oz			▓	25
Oatmeal					
instant (Quaker)	8¾ oz		▓		17

Food	Portion Size	Low GI (0–55)	Mid-GI (56–69)	High GI (70–100)	GL
regular, barley	1¾ oz		■		17
regular, rolled oats	8¾ oz			■	17
Polenta, cooked	8 oz			■	40
Rye	1¾ oz	■			13
Wheat					
bulgur, boiled	1¾ oz	■			12
durum, precooked, cooked 20 minutes	1¾ oz	■			19
semolina, steamed	5¼ oz	■			6
triticum, whole kernels	1¾ oz	■			14
Grape juice	8¾ oz		■		24
Grape leaf, stuffed with rice, lamb, tomato sauce	3½ oz	■			5
Grapefruit	4⅕ oz	■			3
Grapefruit juice, unsweetened	8¾ oz	■			11
Grape-Nuts Flakes cereal (Post)	1 oz			■	17
Grape-Nuts cereal (Post)	1 oz			■	15
Grapes					
dried (raisins)	2 oz		■		28
fresh	4⅕ oz	■			8
Greek foods (_See_ Middle Eastern Foods)					

Food	Portion Size	Low GI (0–55)	Mid-GI (56–69)	High GI (70–100)	GL
Green bell pepper	Standard	Insignificant Carbs			—
Green pea soup (Campbell's)	8³/₄ oz		▓		27
Green peas, frozen	2⁴/₅ oz	▓			3
Greens, collards	Standard	Insignificant Carbs			—
Greens, dandelion	Standard	Insignificant Carbs			—
Greens, leafy (*See* Leafy Greens)					
Greens, mustard	Standard	Insignificant Carbs			—
Greens, turnip	Standard	Insignificant Carbs			—
Ham	Standard	Insignificant Carbs			—
Hamburger bun	1 bun		▓		12
Hamburger patty, 100% meat	Standard	Insignificant Carbs			—
Haricot beans					
baked, canned in tomato sauce	5¹/₄ oz	▓			11
boiled	5¹/₄ oz	▓			9
pressure-cooked	5¹/₄ oz	▓			12
Hazelnuts	Standard	Insignificant Carbs			—
Hellman's mayonnaise	Standard	Insignificant Carbs			—
Honey (*See also* Sweeteners)					
commercial	¹/₃ oz			▓	15
raw	1 oz		▓		10
Honeydew	8 oz	▓			5

Food	Portion Size	Low GI (0–55)	Mid-GI (56–69)	High GI (70–100)	GL
Hot chocolate, made with water (Nestlé)	8¾ oz	▓			1
Hot dog, 100% meat	Standard	Insignificant Carbs			—
Hot dog bun	1 bun		▓		12
Hummus	Standard	Insignificant Carbs			—

ICE CREAM (*See also* Desserts; Frozen non-dairy dessert)					
High-fat (premium)					
chocolate (15% fat)	1¾ oz	▓			4
French vanilla (16% fat)	1¾ oz	▓			3
Low-fat					
chocolate (1.4% fat)	1¾ oz	▓			5
vanilla (1.2% fat)	1¾ oz	▓			5
Regular-fat					
chocolate	1¾ oz		▓		8
half-vanilla, half-chocolate	1¾ oz		▓		8
vanilla	1¾ oz		▓		8

Iceberg lettuce	Standard	Insignificant Carbs			—
Indian bread (*See* Chapatti)					
Instant noodles	2⅔ oz	▓			6

Food	Portion Size	Low GI (0–55)	Mid-GI (56–69)	High GI (70–100)	GL
Ironman PR Bar, chocolate (PR Nutrition)	2¼ oz		■		10

> **TIP**
> When boiling pasta for your favorite Italian dish, keep in mind that, in general, the longer you cook it, the higher the GI will rise. Longer cooking times make pasta quicker and easier to digest, causing blood sugar levels to rise more quickly.

ITALIAN FOODS

Food	Portion Size	Low GI (0–55)	Mid-GI (56–69)	High GI (70–100)	GL
Capellini pasta	6⅓ oz	■			20
Corn pasta, gluten-free	6⅓ oz			■	32
Fettuccine, egg	6⅓ oz	■			15
Gnocchi	6⅓ oz		■		33
Linguine, durum	6⅓ oz	■			23
Pastina	6⅓ oz	■			18
Pizza, cheese					
regular crust	3½ oz		■		16
with tomato sauce, regular crust	3½ oz			■	22
with tomato sauce, thin crust	3½ oz	■			7
with tomato sauce, vegetables, thin crust	3½ oz	■			12
Risotto (boiled Arborio rice)	5¼ oz		■		36

Food	Portion Size	Low GI (0–55)	Mid-GI (56–69)	High GI (70–100)	GL
Sausage, Italian-style	3½ oz	■			1
Spaghetti					
durum, boiled 12 minutes	6⅓ oz	■			21
durum, boiled 20 minutes	6⅓ oz		■		27
white, boiled 5 minutes	6⅓ oz	■			18
whole wheat	6⅓ oz	■			16
with meat sauce, homemade	12½ oz		■		25
Tortellini, cheese	6⅓ oz		■		10
Vermicelli					
durum wheat	5 oz	■			15
white	6⅓ oz	■			16
Italian sausage	3½ oz	■			1
Jalepeño peppers	1 pepper	■			5

JAMS, JELLIES, AND PRESERVES					
Apricot jam	1 oz	■			5
Orange marmalade	1 oz	■			9
Strawberry jam	1 oz	■			10

Japanese foods (*See* Asian Foods)

Food	Portion Size	Low GI (0–55)	Mid-GI (56–69)	High GI (70–100)	GL
Japanese radish (daikon)	Standard	Insignificant Carbs			—
Japanese rice balls (mochi)					
plain	2½ oz	■			14
plain roasted	2½ oz			■	21
salted and roasted	2½ oz			■	20
Jasmine rice, cooked in rice cooker	5¼ oz			■	46
Jelly (*See* Jams, Jellies, and Preserves)					
Jelly beans	1 oz			■	22
JUICES					
Apple, unsweetened	8¾ oz	■			12
Blueberry	8¾ oz		■		14
Carrot, fresh and unsweetened	8¾ oz	■			10
Cranberry, cocktail (Ocean Spray)	8¾ oz			■	24
Grape	8¾ oz		■		24
Grapefruit, unsweetened	8¾ oz	■			11
Orange					
fresh	8¾ oz	■			12
from frozen concentrate	8¾ oz		■		15
unsweetened, reconstituted	8¾ oz	■			9

Food	Portion Size	Low GI (0–55)	Mid-GI (56–69)	High GI (70–100)	GL
Pineapple, unsweetened (Dole)	8¾ oz	■			16
Pomegranate	8¾ oz		■		23
Tomato, unsweetened	8¾ oz	■			4
Kaiser roll	1 oz			■	12
Kale	Standard	Insignificant Carbs			—
Kidney beans, boiled	5¼ oz	■			7
Kiwi	4⅕ oz	■			6
Lactitol (*See also* Sweeteners)	Standard	Insignificant Carbs			—
Lactose (*See also* Sweeteners)	⅓ oz	■			5

FAQ	Why are leafy greens and so many other vegetables not ranked on the glycemic index? (See page 14.)

LEAFY GREENS					
Arugula	Standard	Insignificant Carbs			—
Broccoli rabe (rapini)	Standard	Insignificant Carbs			—
Chicory	Standard	Insignificant Carbs			—
Collard greens	Standard	Insignificant Carbs			—
Dandelion greens	Standard	Insignificant Carbs			—
Endive, Belgian	Standard	Insignificant Carbs			—

Food	Portion Size	Low GI (0–55)	Mid-GI (56–69)	High GI (70–100)	GL
Escarole (Batavia endive)	Standard	Insignificant Carbs			—
Kale	Standard	Insignificant Carbs			—
Lettuce, iceberg	Standard	Insignificant Carbs			—
Lettuce, romaine	Standard	Insignificant Carbs			—
Mustard greens	Standard	Insignificant Carbs			—
Spinach	Standard	Insignificant Carbs			—
Swiss chard	Standard	Insignificant Carbs			—
Turnip greens	Standard	Insignificant Carbs			—
Watercress	Standard	Insignificant Carbs			—
Lebanese bread	1 oz			▓	12
Legumes (*See* Beans and Legumes)					
Lemonade	6 oz		▓		13
Lentil soup	8¾ oz		▓		27
Lentils					
green, boiled	5¼ oz	▓			5
red, boiled	5¼ oz	▓			5
Lettuce (*See also* Leafy Greens)					
iceberg	Standard	Insignificant Carbs			—
romaine	Standard	Insignificant Carbs			—
Life cereal (Quaker Oats)	1 oz		▓		16

Food	Portion Size	Low GI (0–55)	Mid-GI (56–69)	High GI (70–100)	GL
Life Savers (Nestlé)	1 oz				21
Lima beans, boiled (butter beans)					
plain	5¼ oz				6
with sugar added	5¼ oz				6
Linguine pasta, durum	6⅓ oz				23
Linseed rye bread, whole grain	1 oz / 1 slice				7

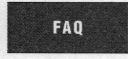

FAQ — Why don't liquor varieties have GI numbers? Aren't they made from high-carbohydrate ingredients? (See page 15.)

LIQUORS			
Bourbon	Standard	Insignificant Carbs	—
Gin	Standard	Insignificant Carbs	—
Rum	Standard	Insignificant Carbs	—
Rye	Standard	Insignificant Carbs	—
Scotch	Standard	Insignificant Carbs	—
Tequila	Standard	Insignificant Carbs	—
Vodka	Standard	Insignificant Carbs	—
Whiskey	Standard	Insignificant Carbs	—
Liver, beef or chicken	Standard	Insignificant Carbs	—

Food	Portion Size	Low GI (0–55)	Mid-GI (56–69)	High GI (70–100)	GL
Liverwurst, 100% meat	Standard	Insignificant Carbs			—
Lobster	Standard	Insignificant Carbs			—
Long-grain rice					
boiled	5¼ oz	▓			22
parboiled and cooked 10 minutes (Uncle Ben's)	5¼ oz				25
parboiled and cooked 20 minutes (Uncle Ben's)	5¼ oz			▓	28

LUNCHEON MEATS, 100% MEAT					
Bologna	Standard	Insignificant Carbs			—
Chicken	Standard	Insignificant Carbs			—
Ham	Standard	Insignificant Carbs			—
Liverwurst	Standard	Insignificant Carbs			—
Pastrami	Standard	Insignificant Carbs			—
Salami	Standard	Insignificant Carbs			—
Turkey	Standard	Insignificant Carbs			—

Food	Portion Size	Low GI (0–55)	Mid-GI (56–69)	High GI (70–100)	GL
Lychees, canned in syrup and drained	4⅕ oz			▓	16
Macadamia nuts	Standard	Insignificant Carbs			—
Macaroni, elbow	6⅓ oz	▓			22
Macaroni and cheese (Kraft)	6⅓ oz		▓		32

Food	Portion Size	Low GI (0–55)	Mid-GI (56–69)	High GI (70–100)	GL
Malt liquor	Standard	Insignificant Carbs			—
Maltose (*See also* Sweeteners)	$\frac{1}{3}$ oz			▓	11
M&M's, Peanut (Mars)	1 oz	▓			6
Mangos	4 oz	▓			8
Margarine	Standard	Insignificant Carbs			—
Marmalade, orange	1 oz	▓			9
Marrowfat peas, boiled	5¼ oz	▓			7
Mars candy bar (Mars)	2 oz		▓		27
Marshmallows	1		▓		5
Mashed potatoes					
instant	5¼ oz			▓	17
regular	5¼ oz			▓	15
Mayonnaise					
Hellman's	Standard	Insignificant Carbs			—
Weight Watchers	Standard	Insignificant Carbs			—
Meat spreads (*See* Pâté)					

MEATS (*See also* Fish; Luncheon Meats; Poultry)					
Beef	Standard	Insignificant Carbs			—
Ham	Standard	Insignificant Carbs			—
Hamburger	Standard	Insignificant Carbs			—

Food	Portion Size	Low GI (0–55)	Mid-GI (56–69)	High GI (70–100)	GL
Liver	Standard	Insignificant Carbs			—
Pork	Standard	Insignificant Carbs			—
Sausage, Italian-style	3½ oz	▓			1
Steak	Standard	Insignificant Carbs			—

Melba toast	1 oz			▓	16

TIP

When shopping for melons, and for fruits in general, you'll want to look for lower-GI selections. Why do some fruits have higher GIs than others? Differences in fiber levels and sugar types are usually to blame. Fruits that are high in fiber and fructose generally have low-GI values, while low-fiber, glucose-rich fruits have higher GI values.

MELONS					
Cantaloupe	4⅕ oz		▓		4
Honeydew	8 oz	▓			5
Watermelon	4⅕ oz			▓	4

Mexican Fast & Fancy rice (Uncle Ben's)	5¼ oz		▓		22

Food	Portion Size	Low GI (0–55)	Mid-GI (56–69)	High GI (70–100)	GL
MEXICAN FOODS					
Beans, boiled					
black	5¼ oz	■			7
brown	5¼ oz	■			9
pinto	5¼ oz	■			10
Mexican Fast & Fancy rice (Uncle Ben's)	5¼ oz		■		22
Peppers, jalapeño	1 pepper		■		5
Taco shell	½ oz		■		11
Tortilla					
corn	1¾ oz	■			12
wheat	1¾ oz	■			8
white	1¾ oz	■			5
Tortilla, corn with refried pinto beans, tomato sauce	3½ oz	■			9
Tortilla, fried corn with mashed potato, tomato, lettuce	3½ oz			■	11
MIDDLE EASTERN FOODS					
Bread, Lebanese	1 oz			■	12
Bread, Turkish					
white-wheat	1 oz			■	15
whole wheat	1 oz	■			8

Food	Portion Size	Low GI (0–55)	Mid-GI (56–69)	High GI (70–100)	GL
Bulgur wheat, boiled	1¾ oz	■			12
Chickpeas, boiled (garbanzo beans)					
in brine	5¼ oz	■			9
in curry	5¼ oz	■			7
plain	5¼ oz	■			9
Couscous	5¼ oz		■		23
Couscous, Moroccan, with semolina, chickpeas, veggies	8¾ oz		■		17
Grape leaf, stuffed with rice, lamb, tomato sauce	3½ oz	■			5
Honey, raw	1 oz	■			10
Hummus	Standard	Insignificant Carbs			—
Pita bread					
wheat	1 oz		■		10
white	1 oz		■		10
Rice					
basmati, boiled white	5¼ oz		■		22
brown, boiled	5¼ oz	■			21
brown, steamed	5¼ oz	■			16
long-grain, boiled	5¼ oz	■			22
white, boiled	5¼ oz		■		25
Soup with Turkish noodles	Standard	Insignificant Carbs			—

Food	Portion Size	Low GI (0–55)	Mid-GI (56–69)	High GI (70–100)	GL
MILK					
Buttermilk	8¾ oz	▨			5
Chocolate	1¾ oz	▨			12
Condensed, sweetened (Nestlé)	1¾ oz		▨		17
Skim	8¾ oz	▨			4
Soy					
full-fat	8¾ oz	▨			8
reduced-fat	8¾ oz	▨			8
Whole	8¾ oz	▨			3
Millet, boiled	5¼ oz			▨	25
Minestrone soup (Campbell's)	8¾ oz	▨			7
Mini-Wheats cereal (Kellogg's)	4 oz		▨		10
Mixers, drink					
Cranberry Juice Cocktail (Ocean Spray)	8¾ oz			▨	24
Orange juice					
fresh	8¾ oz	▨			12
from frozen concentrate	8¾ oz		▨		15
unsweetened, reconstituted	8¾ oz	▨			9
Seltzer	Standard	Insignificant Carbs			—
Tomato juice, unsweetened	8¾ oz	▨			4

Food	Portion Size	Low GI (0–55)	Mid-GI (56–69)	High GI (70–100)	GL
Tonic water (Schweppes)	8¾ oz		■		17
Mochi (*See* Japanese rice balls)					
Mousse (*See* Puddings, Custards, and Mousse)					
Muesli, Alpen, cereal (Weetabix)	1 oz	■			10

MUFFINS					
Apple					
with sugar	2 oz / 1 muffin	■			13
without sugar	2 oz / 1 muffin	■			9
Blueberry	2 oz / 1 muffin		■		17
Bran	2 oz / 1 muffin		■		15
Carrot	2 oz / 1 muffin		■		20
Corn, with low amylose	2 oz / 1 muffin			■	30
English	1 oz / 1 muffin			■	11
Oatmeal	2 oz / 1 muffin			■	24

Multigrain bread					
9-grain	1 oz / 1 slice	■			6
gluten-free	1 oz / 1 slice			■	10
Mung bean noodles	6⅓ oz	■			14
Mung beans					

Food	Portion Size	Low GI (0–55)	Mid-GI (56–69)	High GI (70–100)	GL
boiled	5¼ oz	■			5
pressure-cooked	5¼ oz	■			7
sprouted	5¼ oz	■			4
Mustard	Standard	Insignificant Carbs			—
Mustard greens	Standard	Insignificant Carbs			—
Natural sweeteners (*See* Sweeteners)					
Navy beans					
boiled	5¼ oz	■			9
pressure-cooked	5¼ oz	■			12
Non-dairy dessert, frozen					
tofu-based, chocolate	1¾ oz			■	10
Noodle soup, Turkish	Standard	Insignificant Carbs			—

NOODLES (*See also* Pasta)					
Brown rice	6⅓ oz			■	35
Egg	2⅔ oz	■			5
Instant	2⅔ oz	■			6
Mung bean	6⅓ oz	■			14
Udon, plain	6⅓ oz	■			23
Vermicelli, durum wheat	5 oz	■			15
Vermicelli, white	6⅓ oz	■			16

Food	Portion Size	Low GI (0-55)	Mid-GI (56-69)	High GI (70-100)	GL
White rice	6⅓ oz		■		23

Nopal (cactus pear)	Standard	Insignificant Carbs			—
NutraSweet (aspartame) (*See also* Sweeteners)	Standard	Insignificant Carbs			—

NUTRITIONAL DRINKS					
Choice (Mead Johnson)	7 oz	■			6
Enercal Plus (Wyeth-Ayerst), mix	7 oz		■		24
Ensure (Abbott)	7 oz	■			19
Ensure Plus (Abbott)	4 oz	■			9
Glucerna, vanilla (Abbott)	7 oz	■			7
Ultracal with fiber (Mead Johnson)	7 oz	■			12

NUTS					
Almonds	Standard	Insignificant Carbs			—
Cashews, salted	1¾ oz	■			3
Hazelnuts	Standard	Insignificant Carbs			—
Macadamia	Standard	Insignificant Carbs			—
Peanuts	1¾ oz	■			1
Pecans	Standard	Insignificant Carbs			—

Food	Portion Size	Low GI (0–55)	Mid-GI (56–69)	High GI (70–100)	GL
Walnuts	Standard	Insignificant Carbs			—
Oat bran bread	1 oz / 1 slice	▓			6
Oat Bran cereal (Quaker)	⅓ oz	▓			2
Oatmeal					
Instant (Quaker)	8¾ oz		▓		17
Regular					
barley	1¾ oz		▓		17
rolled oats	8¾ oz			▓	17
Oatmeal cookies	1 oz	▓			9
Oatmeal muffins	2 oz / 1 muffin	▓			24
Oil and vinegar dressing	Standard	Insignificant Carbs			—
Orange juice					
fresh	8¾ oz	▓			12
from frozen concentrate	8¾ oz		▓		15
unsweetened, reconstituted	8¾ oz	▓			9
Orange soda (Fanta)	8¾ oz			▓	23
Oranges	4⅕ oz	▓			5
Oysters	Standard	Insignificant Carbs			—
Pancakes					

Food	Portion Size	Low GI (0–55)	Mid-GI (56–69)	High GI (70–100)	GL
buckwheat, gluten-free, from premix	2²/₃ oz			■	22
plain, from premix	2²/₃ oz		■		39
Papaya (paw paw)	4¹/₅ oz		■		10
Parsnips	2⁴/₅ oz			■	12

FAQ	Why is pasta ranked as a low-glycemic food? (See page 14.)

PASTA					
Brown rice	6¹/₃ oz			■	35
Capellini	6¹/₃ oz	■			20
Corn pasta, gluten-free	6¹/₃ oz			■	32
Egg noodles	2²/₃ oz	■			5
Fettuccine, egg	6¹/₃ oz	■			15
Gnocchi	6¹/₃ oz			■	33
Linguine, durum	6¹/₃ oz	■			23
Macaroni, elbow	6¹/₃ oz	■			22
Macaroni and cheese (Kraft)	6¹/₃ oz		■		32
Mung bean noodles	6¹/₃ oz	■			14
Noodles, instant	2²/₃ oz	■			6
Pastina	6¹/₃ oz	■			18

Food	Portion Size	Low GI (0–55)	Mid-GI (56–69)	High GI (70–100)	GL
Ravioli					
cheese	2⅔ oz	■			15
durum, meat-filled	6⅓ oz	■			15
Rice noodles					
brown	6⅓ oz			■	35
white	6⅓ oz		■		23
Spaghetti					
durum, boiled for 12 minutes	6⅓ oz	■			21
durum, boiled for 20 minutes	6⅓ oz		■		27
white, boiled for 5 minutes	6⅓ oz	■			18
whole wheat	6⅓ oz	■			16
with meat sauce, homemade	12½ oz		■		25
Tortellini, cheese	6⅓ oz		■		10
Udon noodles, plain	6⅓ oz	■			23
Vermicelli					
durum wheat	5 oz	■			15
white	6⅓ oz	■			16
White rice	6⅓ oz		■		23
Pastina	6⅓ oz	■			18
Pastrami	Standard	Insignificant Carbs			—

Food	Portion Size	Low GI (0–55)	Mid-GI (56–69)	High GI (70–100)	GL
Pâté, 100% meat	Standard	Insignificant Carbs			—
Paw paw (papaya)	4⅕ oz		▓		10

TIP	When shopping for peaches or any fruit, choose fresh over canned, and fruits canned in natural juice over more syrupy products. The closer a fruit is to its natural state, the lower its GI is likely to be.

Peaches

Food	Portion Size	Low GI (0–55)	Mid-GI (56–69)	High GI (70–100)	GL
canned in light syrup (Del Monte)	4⅕ oz		▓		9
canned in natural juice	4⅕ oz	▓			5
fresh	4⅕ oz	▓			5
Peanut butter and chocolate chip snack bar (Con Agra)	1⅔ oz	▓			10
Peanut M&M's (Mars)	1 oz	▓			6
Peanuts	1¾ oz	▓			1

Pears

Food	Portion Size	Low GI (0–55)	Mid-GI (56–69)	High GI (70–100)	GL
fresh	4⅕ oz	▓			4
halves, canned in low-sugar syrup	4⅕ oz	▓			4
halves, canned in natural juice	4⅕ oz	▓			5

Food	Portion Size	Low GI (0–55)	Mid-GI (56–69)	High GI (70–100)	GL
PEAS (*See also* Beans and Legumes)					
Black-eyed (cowpeas)	5¼ oz	■			13
Green, frozen	2⅘ oz	■			3
Marrowfat	5¼ oz	■			7
Snap	4 oz / 1 cup	■			10
Split	4 oz	■			6
Pecans	Standard	Insignificant Carbs			—
Peek Frean cookies (Nabisco)	1 oz		■		10
Pepper, black	Standard	Insignificant Carbs			—
Peppers					
green bell	Standard	Insignificant Carbs			—
jalepeño	1 pepper	■			5
red bell	Standard	Insignificant Carbs			—
Pineapple					
canned in syrup	3 oz		■		15
fresh	4⅕ oz		■		7
Pineapple juice, unsweetened (Dole)	8¾ oz	■			16
Pinto beans, boiled					
in brine	5¼ oz	■			4
plain	5¼ oz	■			10

Food	Portion Size	Low GI (0–55)	Mid-GI (56–69)	High GI (70–100)	GL
Pita bread					
wheat	1 oz		■		10
white	1 oz		■		10
Pizza, cheese					
regular crust	3½ oz		■		16
with tomato sauce, regular crust	3½ oz			■	22
with tomato sauce, thin crust	3½ oz	■			7
with tomato sauce, vegetables, thin crust	3½ oz	■			12
Plums					
dried, pitted (prunes)	4⅕ oz	■			6
fresh	4⅕ oz	■			5
Polenta, cooked	8 oz			■	40
Pomegranate juice	8¾ oz		■		23
Pop, soda (*See* Soft Drinks)					
Pop Tarts (Kellogg's)	1 pastry			■	25
Popcorn, plain microwavable	1 oz		■		8
Pork	Standard	Insignificant Carbs			—
Porridge (*See* Oatmeal)					
Potato chips, plain salted	1¾ oz	■			11
Potato crisps (*See* Potato chips)					

Food	Portion Size	Low GI (0-55)	Mid-GI (56-69)	High GI (70-100)	GL
FAQ	How is it possible that a plain baked potato has a higher GI value than potato chips? (See page 13.)				

POTATOES					
Baked, plain russet	5¼ oz			▓	26
Boiled					
plain new	5¼ oz		▓		12
plain white	5¼ oz		▓		14
Canned	5¼ oz			▓	11
French-fried	5¼ oz			▓	22
Mashed	5¼ oz			▓	15
Mashed, instant	5¼ oz			▓	17
Microwaved	5¼ oz			▓	27
Steamed	5¼ oz		▓		20
Sweet	5¼ oz		▓		17

POULTRY (*See also* Fish; Luncheon Meats; Meats)					
Chicken					
nuggets, microwavable	3½ oz	▓			7
parts	Standard	Insignificant Carbs			—
roll, 100% meat	Standard	Insignificant Carbs			—

Food	Portion Size	Low GI (0–55)	Mid-GI (56–69)	High GI (70–100)	GL
Duck	Standard	Insignificant Carbs			—
Goose	Standard	Insignificant Carbs			—
Turkey	Standard	Insignificant Carbs			—
Pound cake	2 oz	■			15
Power Bar (Powerfood)	2¼ oz		■		24
Preserves (*See* Jams, Jellies, and Preserves)					
Pretzels, wheat	1 oz			■	16
Prunes, pitted	4⅕ oz	■			6

PUDDINGS, CUSTARDS, AND MOUSSE					
Custard, homemade, with milk	3½ oz	■			7
Mousse, instant reduced-fat, with water	1¾ oz	■			4
Pudding, chocolate, from premix	4 oz	■			10
Pudding, instant, with whole milk	3½ oz	■			7
Pudding, Tapioca, with milk	4½ oz			■	40
Pudding, vanilla, from premix	4 oz	■			9

Puffed Wheat cereal (Quaker)	1 oz		■		13
Pumpernickel bread, whole grain	1 oz / 1 slice	■			5

Food	Portion Size	Low GI (0–55)	Mid-GI (56–69)	High GI (70–100)	GL
Pumpkin	3⅔ oz			■	5
Quik, chocolate (Nestlé)					
made with 1.5%-fat milk	8¾ oz	■			5
made with water	8¾ oz	■			4
Quik, strawberry (Nestlé)					
made with 1.5%-fat milk	8¾ oz	■			4
made with water	8¾ oz		■		5
Rabe, broccoli (rapini)	Standard	Insignificant Carbs			—
Radicchio (red chicory)	Standard	Insignificant Carbs			—
Radish, Chinese	Standard	Insignificant Carbs			—
Radish, daikon	Standard	Insignificant Carbs			—
Raisin Bran cereal (Kellogg's)	1 oz		■		12
Raisin bread	1 oz / 1 slice	■			10
Raisins	2 oz		■		28
Rapini (broccoli rabe)	Standard	Insignificant Carbs			—
Raspberries	8 oz	■			5
Raspberry smoothie drink	8¾ oz	■			14
Ravioli					
cheese	2⅔ oz	■			15
durum, meat-filled	6⅓ oz	■			15
Red bell pepper	Standard	Insignificant Carbs			—

Food	Portion Size	Low GI (0–55)	Mid-GI (56–69)	High GI (70–100)	GL
Red leaf chicory (radicchio)	Standard	Insignificant Carbs			—
Red River Cereal (Maple Leaf Mills)	1 oz	▓			11

FAQ	Why do different rice varieties have different GI rankings? (See page 12.)

RICE					
Arborio, boiled (risotto)	5¼ oz		▓		36
Basmati, white					
boiled	5¼ oz	▓			22
microwaved in pouch (Uncle Ben's)	5¼ oz	▓			24
quick-cooking, cooked 10 minutes (Uncle Ben's)	5¼ oz	▓			23
Brown					
boiled	5¼ oz		▓		21
parboiled and cooked 20 minutes (Uncle Ben's)	5¼ oz		▓		23
steamed	5¼ oz	▓			16
Cajun Style (Uncle Ben's)	5¼ oz		▓		19
Curry	5¼ oz		▓		41
Curry, with cheese	5¼ oz	▓			27
Garden Style (Uncle Ben's)	5¼ oz	▓			21

Food	Portion Size	Low GI (0–55)	Mid-GI (56–69)	High GI (70–100)	GL
Jasmine, cooked in rice cooker	5¼ oz			■	46
Long-grain					
boiled	5¼ oz	■	■		22
converted, parboiled 25 minutes (Uncle Ben's)	5¼ oz	■			18
parboiled and cooked 10 minutes (Uncle Ben's)	5¼ oz		■		25
parboiled and cooked 20 minutes (Uncle Ben's)	5¼ oz		■		28
Mexican Fast & Fancy (Uncle Ben's)	5¼ oz		■		22
Saskatchewan wild rice	5¼ oz		■		18
Sticky rice (glutinous rice)	5¼ oz			■	44
White					
boiled	5¼ oz		■		25
converted, parboiled 25 minutes (Uncle Ben's)	5¼ oz	■			14
instant, boiled 1 minute	5¼ oz	■			19
parboiled (Canada)	5¼ oz	■			18
parboiled (US)	5¼ oz			■	26
with butter	5¼ oz			■	40
Rice balls, Japanese (mochi)					
plain	2½ oz	■			14
plain roasted	2½ oz	■			21

Food	Portion Size	Low GI (0–55)	Mid-GI (56–69)	High GI (70–100)	GL
salted and roasted	2½ oz			■	20
Rice cakes	1 oz			■	17
Rice Chex cereal (Nabisco)	1 oz			■	23
Rice crackers, plain (sembei)	1 oz			■	23
Rice Krispies cereal (Kellogg's)	1 oz			■	21
Rice noodles					
brown	6⅓ oz			■	35
white	6⅓ oz		■		23
Rich Tea cookies	1 oz	■			10
Risotto (boiled Arborio rice)	5¼ oz		■		36

ROLLS (*See also* Breads)					
Croissants	2 oz		■		17
Hamburger buns	1 bun		■		12
Frankfurter buns	1 bun		■		12
Kaiser rolls	1 oz			■	12
Scones, plain, from premix	1 oz			■	8

Romaine lettuce	Standard	Insignificant Carbs			—
Romano beans, boiled	4 oz	■			8

Food	Portion Size	Low GI (0–55)	Mid-GI (56–69)	High GI (70–100)	GL

TIP	When choosing potatoes, consider buying sweet potatoes rather than the usual white varieties. Because a white potato provides a rapidly digestible starch and has virtually no fiber, it's a high-GI choice. Sweet potatoes have a lower GI ranking because they're rich in fiber.

ROOT VEGETABLES

Potatoes

Food	Portion Size	Low GI (0–55)	Mid-GI (56–69)	High GI (70–100)	GL
baked, plain russet	5¼ oz			▓	26
boiled, plain new	5¼ oz		▓		12
boiled, plain white	5¼ oz				14
canned	5¼ oz		▓		11
French-fried	5¼ oz			▓	22
mashed	5¼ oz			▓	15
mashed, instant	5¼ oz			▓	17
microwaved	5¼ oz			▓	27
steamed	5¼ oz		▓		20
Sweet potatoes	5¼ oz		▓		17
Taro	5¼ oz		▓		4
Yams	5¼ oz	▓			13

Food	Portion Size	Low GI (0–55)	Mid-GI (56–69)	High GI (70–100)	GL
Rum (liquor)	Standard	Insignificant Carbs			—
Rutabaga (swede)	5¼ oz		■		7
Rye (grain)	1¾ oz	■			13
Rye (liquor)	Standard	Insignificant Carbs			—
Rye bread					
cocktail	1 oz / 1 slice	■			7
kernel	1 oz / 1 slice	■			5
light	1 oz / 1 slice		■		10
linseed, whole grain	1 oz / 1 slice	■			8
sourdough	1 oz / 1 slice	■			6
whole grain	1 oz / 1 slice		■		8
Salad dressing					
oil and vinegar	Standard	Insignificant Carbs			—
Salami, 100% meat	Standard	Insignificant Carbs			—
Salt	Standard	Insignificant Carbs			—
Saskatchewan wild rice	5¼ oz		■		18
Sausage, Italian-style	3½ oz	■			1
Scallops	Standard	Insignificant Carbs			—
Scones, plain, from premix	1 oz			■	8
Scotch (liquor)	Standard	Insignificant Carbs			—

Food	Portion Size	Low GI (0–55)	Mid-GI (56–69)	High GI (70–100)	GL
SEAFOOD (*See also* Fish)					
Clams	Standard	Insignificant Carbs			—
Crabmeat	Standard	Insignificant Carbs			—
Lobster	Standard	Insignificant Carbs			—
Oysters	Standard	Insignificant Carbs			—
Scallops	Standard	Insignificant Carbs			—
Shrimp	Standard	Insignificant Carbs			—
Seltzer	Standard	Insignificant Carbs			—
Sembei (rice crackers)	1 oz			■	23
Semolina, steamed	5¼ oz	■			6
Shredded Wheat cereal (Nabisco)	1 oz		■		15
Shrimp	Standard	Insignificant Carbs			—
Skim	8¾ oz	■			
Skittles (Mars)	1⅔ oz		■		32
Smoothie drinks					
banana, soy	8¾ oz	■			7
raspberry (Con Agra)	8¾ oz	■			14
Snack bars (*See also* Energy bars; Fruit bars)					
apple cinnamon (Con Agra)	1⅔ oz	■			12

Food	Portion Size	Low GI (0–55)	Mid-GI (56–69)	High GI (70–100)	GL
peanut butter and chocolate chip (Con Agra)	1²/₃ oz	■			10

SNACK FOODS (*See also* Desserts)

Food	Portion Size	Low GI (0–55)	Mid-GI (56–69)	High GI (70–100)	GL
Apple cinnamon bar (Con Agra)	1²/₃ oz	■			12
Corn chips, salted	1³/₄ oz		■		17
Peanut butter and chocolate chip bar (Con Agra)	1²/₃ oz	■			10
Pop Tarts (Kellogg's)	1 pastry			■	25
Popcorn, plain microwavable	1 oz			■	8
Potato chips, plain salted	1³/₄ oz	■			11
Pretzels, wheat	1 oz			■	16
Tortilla chips	1³/₄ oz		■		17
Snap peas, boiled	4 oz / 1 cup	■			10
Snickers candy bar (Mars)	2 oz		■		23
Soba noodle soup, instant	6¹/₃ oz	■			22
Soda pop (*See* Soft Drinks)					
Soda Crackers, Premium (Christie Brown & Co.)	1 oz			■	12

SOFT DRINKS

Cola (Coca-Cola)

Food	Portion Size	Low GI (0–55)	Mid-GI (56–69)	High GI (70–100)	GL
Diet Coke	Standard	Insignificant Carbs			—
regular Coke	12 oz		■		16
Orange (Fanta)	8¾ oz			■	23
Seltzer	Standard	Insignificant Carbs			—
Tonic water (Schweppes)	8¾ oz		■		17

SOUPS					
Black bean	8¾ oz		■		17
Green pea (Campbell's)	8¾ oz		■		27
Lentil	8¾ oz	■			9
Minestrone (Campbell's)	8¾ oz	■			7
Noodle, Turkish	Standard	Insignificant Carbs			—
Soba noodle, instant	6⅓ oz		■		22
Split pea	8¾ oz		■		16
Tomato	8¾ oz	■			6

Sour cream	Standard	Insignificant Carbs			—
Sourdough bread					
rye	1 oz / 1 slice	■			6
wheat	1 oz / 1 slice	■			6
Soy and linseed bread	1 oz / 1 slice	■			6

Food	Portion Size	Low GI (0–55)	Mid-GI (56–69)	High GI (70–100)	GL
Soy beans	5¼ oz	■			1
Soy products					
Flour	8 oz	■			10
Milk					
reduced-fat	8¾ oz	■			8
whole (full-fat)	8¾ oz	■			8
Smoothie, banana	8¾ oz	■			7
Yogurt, reduced-fat	7 oz	■			13
Spaghetti (*See also* Pasta)					
durum, boiled 12 minutes	6⅓ oz	■			21
durum, boiled 20 minutes	6⅓ oz		■		27
white, boiled 5 minutes	6⅓ oz	■			18
whole wheat	6⅓ oz	■			16
with meat sauce, homemade	12½ oz		■		25
Special K cereal (Kellogg's)	1 oz		■		14
Spinach	Standard	Insignificant Carbs			—
Spirits (*See* Liquors)					
Splenda (sucralose) (*See also* Sweeteners)	Standard	Insignificant Carbs			—
Split pea soup	8¾ oz		■		16
Split peas, boiled	4 oz	■			6
Sponge cake	2⅕ oz	■			17

Food	Portion Size	Low GI (0–55)	Mid-GI (56–69)	High GI (70–100)	GL
Sports bars (*See* Energy bars)					
Sports drinks (*See also* Nutritional Drinks)					
Gatorade	8 3/4 oz			░	12
SPREADS					
Apricot jam	1 oz	░			5
Butter	Standard	Insignificant Carbs			—
Hummus	Standard	Insignificant Carbs			—
Margarine	Standard	Insignificant Carbs			—
Marmalade, orange	1 oz	░			9
Mayonnaise					
Hellman's	Standard	Insignificant Carbs			—
Weight Watchers	Standard	Insignificant Carbs			—
Pâté, 100% meat	Standard	Insignificant Carbs			—
Spelt bread					
multigrain	1 oz / 1 slice	░			7
white	1 oz / 1 slice			░	17
whole grain	1 oz / 1 slice		░		12
Split peas, boiled	4 oz	░			6
Sprouts, Brussels	Standard	Insignificant Carbs			—

Food	Portion Size	Low GI (0–55)	Mid-GI (56–69)	High GI (70–100)	GL
Squash					
acorn	4 oz			▓	10
butternut	4 oz			▓	10
zucchini	Standard	Insignificant Carbs			—
Steak (*See also* Meats)	Standard	Insignificant Carbs			—
Stevia (*See also* Sweeteners)	Standard	Insignificant Carbs			—
Sticky rice (glutinous rice)	5¼ oz			▓	44
Stoned Wheat Thins (Christie Brown & Co.)	1 oz		▓		12
Strawberries	4⅕ oz	▓			1
Strawberry jam	1 oz	▓			10
Strawberry Quik (Nestlé)					
made with 1.5%-fat milk	8¾ oz	▓			4
made with water	8¾ oz		▓		5
Sucralose (*See also* Sweeteners)	Standard	Insignificant Carbs			—
Sucrose (*See also* Sweeteners)	⅓ oz		▓		10

FAQ	Why isn't sugar ranked high on the GI? (See page 14.)

| **Sugar** (*See also* Sweeteners) | ½ oz | | ▓ | | 8 |
| **Sultanas** (*See* Raisins) | | | | | |

Food	Portion Size	Low GI (0–55)	Mid-GI (56–69)	High GI (70–100)	GL
Sushi					
salmon	3½ oz		▓		17
sea algae, roasted with vinegar and rice	3½ oz	▓			20
Swede (rutabaga)	5¼ oz		▓		7
Sweet corn					
canned, diet pack	2⅘ oz	▓			7
frozen, microwavable	2⅘ oz	▓			7
on cob, boiled 20 minutes	2⅘ oz		▓		11
Sweet potatoes	5¼ oz		▓		17
SWEETENERS					
Blue agave cactus, organic, high-fructose (Western Commerce)	⅓ oz	▓			1
Fructose	⅓ oz	▓			1
Glucose	⅓ oz			▓	10
Honey					
commercial	⅓ oz			▓	15
raw	1 oz		▓		10
Lactitol	Standard	Insignificant Carbs			—
Lactose	⅓ oz	▓			5
Maltose	⅓ oz			▓	11
NutraSweet (aspartame)	Standard	Insignificant Carbs			—

Food	Portion Size	Low GI (0–55)	Mid-GI (56–69)	High GI (70–100)	GL
Splenda (sucralose)	Standard	Insignificant Carbs			—
Stevia	Standard	Insignificant Carbs			—
Sucrose	⅓ oz		▓		10
Sugar	½ oz		▓		8
Xylitol	⅓ oz	▓			1
Swiss chard	Standard	Insignificant Carbs			—
Taco shell	½ oz		▓		11
Tapioca	4 oz			▓	14
Tapioca pudding with milk	4½ oz			▓	40
Taro	5¼ oz		▓		4
Tea	Standard	Insignificant Carbs			—
Tea cookies, Rich	1 oz	▓			10
Team Flakes cereal (Nabisco)	1 oz			▓	17
Tequila (liquor)	Standard	Insignificant Carbs			—
Thai foods (*See* Asian Foods)					
Toast, melba	1 oz			▓	16
Tofu	Standard	Insignificant Carbs			—

TIP	Looking for a packaged food that isn't listed? Estimate the product's GI by following the guidelines presented on page 20.

Food	Portion Size	Low GI (0–55)	Mid-GI (56–69)	High GI (70–100)	GL
Tofu frozen dessert	1¾ oz			■	10
Tomato, fresh	1 medium	■			1
Tomato juice, unsweetened	8¾ oz	■			4
Tomato soup	8¾ oz	■			6
Tonic water (Schweppes)	8¾ oz		■		17
Tortellini, cheese	6⅓ oz		■		10
Tortilla, corn with refried pinto beans, tomato sauce	3½ oz	■			9
Tortilla, fried corn with mashed potato, tomato, lettuce	3½ oz			■	11
Tortilla chips	1¾ oz		■		17
Tortillas					
corn	1¾ oz	■			12
wheat	1¾ oz	■			8
white	1¾ oz	■			5
Total cereal (General Mills)	1 oz			■	17
Triticum wheat, whole kernels	1¾ oz	■			14
Turkey					
parts	Standard	Insignificant Carbs			—
roll, 100% meat	Standard	Insignificant Carbs			—
Turkish bread					

Food	Portion Size	Low GI (0–55)	Mid-GI (56–69)	High GI (70–100)	GL
white-wheat	1 oz / 1 slice			▓	15
whole wheat	1 oz / 1 slice	▓			8

Turkish foods (*See* Middle Eastern Foods)

Food	Portion Size	Low GI (0–55)	Mid-GI (56–69)	High GI (70–100)	GL
Turkish noodle soup	Standard	Insignificant Carbs			—
Turnip greens	Standard	Insignificant Carbs			—
Twix candy bar (Mars)	2 oz	▓			17
Ultracal nutritional drink with fiber (Mead Johnson)	7 oz	▓			12
Vanilla cake with frosting	4 oz	▓			24

Vanilla ice cream

Food	Portion Size	Low GI (0–55)	Mid-GI (56–69)	High GI (70–100)	GL
high-fat French vanilla (16% fat)	1¾ oz	▓			3
low-fat (1.2% fat)	1¾ oz	▓			5
regular-fat	1¾ oz		▓		8
Vanilla pudding, from premix	4 oz	▓			9

VEGETABLE JUICES					
Carrot, fresh and unsweetened	8¾ oz	▓			10
Tomato, unsweetened	8¾ oz	▓			4

VEGETABLES					
Artichokes	Standard	Insignificant Carbs			—

Food	Portion Size	Low GI (0–55)	Mid-GI (56–69)	High GI (70–100)	GL
Arugula	Standard	Insignificant Carbs			—
Avocados	Standard	Insignificant Carbs			—
Batavia endive (escarole)	Standard	Insignificant Carbs			—
Beets (beetroot)	2⁴/₅ oz		▓		5
Bok choy	Standard	Insignificant Carbs			—
Broccoli	Standard	Insignificant Carbs			—
Broccoli rabe (rapini)	Standard	Insignificant Carbs			—
Brussels sprouts	Standard	Insignificant Carbs			—
Cabbage	Standard	Insignificant Carbs			—
Carrots					
cooked	2²/₃ oz		▓		5
fresh	2⁴/₅ oz			▓	5
Cassava, boiled	2⁴/₅ oz	▓			12
Cauliflower	Standard	Insignificant Carbs			—
Celery	Standard	Insignificant Carbs			—
Chicory	Standard	Insignificant Carbs			—
Collard greens	Standard	Insignificant Carbs			—
Corn, sweet					

FAQ	Why are so many vegetables not ranked on the glycemic index? (See page 14.)

Food	Portion Size	Low GI (0–55)	Mid-GI (56–69)	High GI (70–100)	GL
canned, diet pack	2⅘ oz	■			7
frozen, microwavable	2⅘ oz	■			7
on cob, boiled 20 minutes	2⅘ oz		■	11	
Cucumbers	Standard	Insignificant Carbs			—
Daikon radish (Chinese)	Standard	Insignificant Carbs			—
Dandelion greens	Standard	Insignificant Carbs			—
Endive, Belgian (witloof)	Standard	Insignificant Carbs			—
Escarole (Batavia endive)	Standard	Insignificant Carbs			—
Kale	Standard	Insignificant Carbs			—
Lettuce, iceberg	Standard	Insignificant Carbs			—
Lettuce, romaine	Standard	Insignificant Carbs			—
Mustard greens	Standard	Insignificant Carbs			—
Parsnips	2⅘ oz			■	12
Peppers					
green bell	Standard	Insignificant Carbs			—
Jalepeño	1 pepper	■			5
red bell	Standard	Insignificant Carbs			—
Potatoes					
baked, plain russet	5¼ oz			■	26
boiled, plain new	5¼ oz		■		12
boiled, plain white	5¼ oz		■		14

Food	Portion Size	Low GI (0–55)	Mid-GI (56–69)	High GI (70–100)	GL
canned	5¼ oz		■		11
French-fried	5¼ oz			■	22
mashed	5¼ oz			■	15
mashed, instant	5¼ oz			■	17
microwaved	5¼ oz			■	27
steamed	5¼ oz			■	20
Pumpkin	3⅔ oz			■	5
Radicchio (red chicory)	Standard	Insignificant Carbs			—
Rapini (broccoli rabe)	Standard	Insignificant Carbs			—
Rutabaga (swede)	5¼ oz			■	7
Spinach	Standard	Insignificant Carbs			—
Squash	Standard	Insignificant Carbs			—
Sweet potatoes	5¼ oz		■		17
Swiss chard	Standard	Insignificant Carbs			—
Taro	5¼ oz		■		4
Tomatoes	1 medium	■			1
Turnip greens	Standard	Insignificant Carbs			—
Watercress	Standard	Insignificant Carbs			—
Witloof (Belgian endive)	Standard	Insignificant Carbs			—
Yams	5¼ oz	■			13

Food	Portion Size	Low GI (0–55)	Mid-GI (56–69)	High GI (70–100)	GL
Vermicelli pasta					
durum wheat	5 oz / 1 cup	■			15
white	6⅓ oz	■			16
Vodka (liquor)	Standard	Insignificant Carbs			—
Wafers					
Graham (Christie Brown & Co.)	1 oz			■	14
Vanilla (Christie Brown & Co.)	1 oz			■	14
Waffles	1¼ oz			■	10
Walnuts	Standard	Insignificant Carbs			—
Watercress	Standard	Insignificant Carbs			—
Watermelon	4⅕ oz			■	4
Weetabix cereal (Weetabix)	1 oz		■		16
Weight Watchers mayonnaise	Standard	Insignificant Carbs			—
Weiners (*See* Frankfurters)					
Wheat					
bulgur, boiled	1¾ oz	■			12
durum, precooked, cooked 20 minutes	1¾ oz	■			19
semolina, steamed	5¼ oz	■			6
triticum, whole kernels	1¾ oz	■			14
Wheat bread					

Food	Portion Size	Low GI (0–55)	Mid-GI (56–69)	High GI (70–100)	GL
chapatti	2 oz		■		21
coarse kernel	1 oz / 1 slice	■			10
sourdough	1 oz / 1 slice	■			6
whole wheat, 100%	1 oz / 1 slice			■	10
Wheat crackers, Breton (Dare)	1 oz				10
Wheat pretzels	1 oz				16
Wheat Thins (Nabisco)	8 crackers		■		7
Whiskey (liquor)	Standard	Insignificant Carbs			—
White bread					
gluten-free	1 oz / 1 slice			■	11
regular (Wonder)	1 oz / 1 slice			■	10
whole wheat	1 oz / 1 slice			■	10
White rice					
boiled	5¼ oz		■		25
converted, parboiled 25 minutes (Uncle Ben's)	5¼ oz	■			14
instant, boiled 1 minute	5¼ oz		■		19
long-grain, converted, parboiled 25 min (Uncle Ben's)	5¼ oz	■			18
parboiled (Canada)	5¼ oz		■		18
parboiled (US)	5¼ oz			■	26
with butter	5¼ oz		■		40

Food	Portion Size	Low GI (0–55)	Mid-GI (56–69)	High GI (70–100)	GL
Whole grain bread	1 oz / 1 slice	■			5
Whole wheat bread	1 oz / 1 slice			■	10
Wild rice, Saskatchewan	5¼ oz		■		18

FAQ	Since wine contains an insignificant amount of carbs, can I drink as much as I want? (See pages 15 and 16.)

Food	Portion Size				
Wine					
red	Standard	Insignificant Carbs			—
white	Standard	Insignificant Carbs			—
Witloof (Belgian endive)	Standard	Insignificant Carbs			—
Xylitol (*See also* Sweeteners)	⅓ oz	■			1
Yam	5¼ oz		■		13

YOGURT					
Milk					
low-fat, plain, no sugar	6 oz	■			5
low-fat, with artificial sweetener	7 oz	■			2
low-fat, with sugar	7 oz		■		10
non-fat, with artificial sweetener	7 oz	■			3

Food	Portion Size	Low GI (0–55)	Mid-GI (56–69)	High GI (70–100)	GL
reduced-fat, with fruit	7 oz	■			7
whole, no sugar	7 oz	■			3
Soy-based, reduced fat	7 oz	■			13

| Zucchini | Standard | Insignificant Carbs | | | — |

GLOSSARY

Adult onset diabetes. *See* Type II diabetes.

Blood glucose level. Also called blood sugar level, this is the amount of glucose in the blood at any given time. *See also* High blood sugar; Low blood sugar.

Blood sugar level. *See* Blood glucose level.

Carbohydrates. The body's main and most efficient source of fuel, the other two sources being fat and protein. Carbohydrates are molecules formed by carbon, hydrogen, and oxygen, and can be broken into two main categories—simple and complex. Complex carbohydrates can be further broken into two subcategories—digestible carbohydrates, or starch; and indigestible carbohydrates, or fiber. *See also* Complex carbohydrates; Digestible carbohydrates; Indigestible carbohydrates; Simple carbohydrates.

Cardiovascular disease. A class of diseases that involve the heart and/or blood vessels. This class includes, but is not limited to, arteriosclerosis, coronary artery disease, arrhythmia, hypertension, and congenital heart disease.

Complex carbohydrates. A form of carbohydrate made of chains of hundreds or thousands of simple carbohydrates that have been bonded together. Containing both indigestible and digestible carbohydrates (fiber and starch), complex carbohydrates are metabolized slowly, and therefore do not cause a rapid rise in blood glucose levels. *See also* Digestible carbohydrates; Indigestible carbohydrates; Simple carbohydrates.

Diabetes. *See* Type II diabetes.

Digestible carbohydrates. The subcategory of complex carbohydrates that, as the name implies, can be processed by the human digestive system and used as fuel. Digestible carbohydrates are also known as starch.

Fiber. *See* Indigestible carbohydrates.

Glucose. A simple sugar that is the main source of energy for the body. It is obtained through the breakdown of food during the digestive process, and is carried to each cell via the bloodstream.

Glycemic index (GI). A system developed to rank carbohydrate-rich foods according to their effect on blood glucose levels. Created in 1981 by Dr. David J. Jenkins at the University of Toronto, originally to help diabetes patients manage their blood sugar levels, it signifies how quickly a food triggers a rise in blood glucose (blood sugar). Foods with a GI number of 55 or less are considered low glycemic, meaning that they affect blood sugar levels slowly. Foods that fall between 56 to 69 are in the medium range. Foods with a GI number of 70 or more are considered high glycemic, meaning that they cause a rapid surge in blood sugar levels.

Glycemic load (GL). A system developed to rank carbohydrate-rich foods based on both their glycemic index and the amount being eaten. It is determined by multiplying the food's glycemic index by the grams of carbohydrates contained in the portion, and then dividing it by 100. A GL of 20 or more is considered high; a GL between 11 and 19 is considered moderate; and a GL of 10 or less is considered low.

High blood sugar. A blood level of the sugar glucose that is overly high. This condition is also called hyperglycemia.

High-density lipoprotein (HDL). The so-called "good" cholesterol that collects cholesterol from the body's tissues and transports it to the liver for processing.

Hypertension. Abnormally elevated (high) blood pressure.

Indigestible carbohydrates. The subcategory of complex carbohydrates that cannot be absorbed by the human digestive system, and therefore cannot be used as fuel. Nevertheless, indigestible carbohydrates—often called fiber—have many healthful properties, including the ability to slow the digestive process and thereby help regulate blood glucose levels.

Insulin. A hormone that regulates the level of sugar in the blood. When blood glucose levels rise, the pancreas secretes insulin, which then allows glucose to be transported to and taken in by the cells.

Insulin resistance. A condition in which the cells do not respond properly to insulin, and therefore will not remove and use glucose from the blood. This results in chronically high levels of both insulin and blood sugar, and can spiral into type II diabetes. Insulin resistance is also one of the symptoms of metabolic syndrome. *See* Metabolic syndrome; Type II diabetes.

Low blood sugar. A blood level of the sugar glucose that is too low to meet the body's needs. This condition is also called hypoglycemia.

Low-density lipoprotein (LDL). The so-called "bad" cholesterol that transports cholesterol to the cells of the body.

Metabolic syndrome. A cluster of symptoms that include insulin resistance, hypertension (high blood pressure), high cholesterol, high triglycerides, and increased weight. People with this disorder have been found to be at increased risk for coronary heart disease, stroke, and diabetes. This disorder is sometimes called syndrome X.

Net carbs. The total carbohydrate amount in a food that can be absorbed and digested, and that therefore can affect blood glucose levels and stimulate the production of insulin.

Non-insulin-dependent diabetes. *See* Type II diabetes.

Obesity. The condition of being extremely overweight. This is sometimes defined as being 20 percent over ideal weight, and sometimes defined as having a body mass index (BMI) of 30 or more.

Simple carbohydrates. A form of carbohydrate made

of only one, two, or three units of sugar (saccharide units). Simple carbohydrates are metabolized quickly, causing a surge in blood glucose levels. They are sometimes referred to as simple sugars.

Simple sugars. *See* Simple carbohydrates.

Starch. *See* Digestible carbohydrates.

Syndrome X. *See* Metabolic syndrome.

Triglycerides. The substance that is the main component of animal fat. High levels of triglycerides in the bloodstream are associated with atherosclerosis—the clogging, narrowing, and hardening of the arteries that can lead to heart attack and stroke.

Type II diabetes. A chronic progressive disorder in which the body's cells fail to take up glucose from the bloodstream, causing a high level of sugar in the blood. This disorder, which accounts for about 90 percent of all diabetics, is also referred to as adult onset diabetes and non-insulin-dependent diabetes.

HELPFUL WEBSITES

The glycemic index is a relatively new concept, and more information on the GI is becoming available all the time. Several websites now offer constantly growing databases and lists of foods, their glycemic index, and their glycemic load, as well as practical information that can help you manage your diet and meet your health goals. The following list will get you started, but more websites are sure to appear as further research is performed on this exciting subject.

The Center for Naturopathic Medicine

Website: www.centerfornaturopathic.com

This site provides a concise definition of the glycemic index plus a substantial glycemic index database of foods. Information on a wide range of health concerns is also offered, with an emphasis on nutrition, herbs, and other natural treatments.

Glycemic Index

Website: www.glycemicindex.com

Based in the Human Nutrition Unit of the University of Sydney in Australia, this website is updated by the university's GI group. It includes comprehensive information on the glycemic index, GI testing, and related topics, as well as an extensive international GI database of foods.

The Glycemic Index Foundation of South Africa

Website: www.gifoundation.com

Designed to help people manage their blood glucose levels, this site explains the glycemic index, helps you understand the relationship between GI and glycemic load, and guides you in using these concepts to manage your diet. An extensive list of foods showing GI and GL is included.

Mendosa.com

Website: www.mendosa.com

Created by a medical writer and diabetes specialist, Mendosa.com provides a good deal of information on diabetes management in general, and the glycemic index in particular. Included is a table of international foods that states both the glycemic index and glycemic load of each listed item.

Nutrition Data

Website: www.nutritiondata.com

Click on "Topics" and then "Glycemic Index," and you'll find a wealth of information on the glycemic index, glycemic load, and more. The site also offers more general nutritional information and enables you to access a nutritional analysis of various foods.

Recipe Nutrition

Website: www.recipenutrition.com

In an effort to help individuals meet their dietary needs, Recipe Nutrition provides nutritional information on a number of foods, meals, and various meal plans. Included are recommended food substitutions for switching to a low-glycemic index diet.

ABOUT THE AUTHOR

Dr. Shari Lieberman earned her PhD in Clinical Nutrition and Exercise Physiology from The Union Institute, Cincinnati, Ohio, and her Master of Science degree in Nutrition, Food Science and Dietetics from New York University. She is a Certified Nutrition Specialist (CNS); a Fellow of the American College of Nutrition (FACN); a member of the New York Academy of Science and the American Academy of Anti-Aging Medicine (A4M); a former officer and present board member of the Certification Board for Nutrition Specialists; and President of the American Association for Health Freedom. She is the recipient of the National Nutritional Foods Association 2003 Clinician of the Year Award and a member of the Nutrition Team for the New York City Marathon. Dr. Lieberman is the author of the best-selling *The Real Vitamin & Mineral Book; User's Guide to Brain-Boosting Supplements; Dare to Lose: 4 Simple Steps to a Better Body; Get Off the Menopause Roller Coaster; Maitake Mushroom and D-fraction; Maitake King of Mushrooms;* and *All About Vitamin C.*

Dr. Lieberman is also the Founding Dean of New York Chiropractic College's MS Degree in

Clinical Nutrition, contributing editor to the American Medical Associations' 5th Edition of *Drug Evaluations*, peer reviewer for scientific publications, published scientific researcher, and presenter at numerous scientific conferences. A frequent guest on television and radio programs as an authority on nutrition, Dr. Lieberman has been in private practice as a clinical nutritionist for over twenty years. You can visit her website at *www.drshari.net*.

INDEX

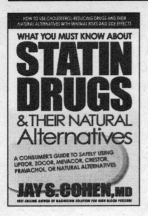

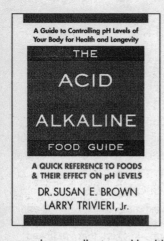

A Guide to Controlling pH Levels of
Your Body for Health and Longevity

THE
ACID
ALKALINE
FOOD GUIDE

A QUICK REFERENCE TO FOODS
& THEIR EFFECT ON pH LEVELS

DR. SUSAN E. BROWN
LARRY TRIVIERI, Jr.

THE ACID-ALKALINE FOOD GUIDE
A Quick Reference to Foods & Their Effect on pH Levels

Susan E. Brown, PhD, CCN
and Larry Trivieri, Jr.

In the last few years, researchers around the world have reported the importance of acid-alkaline balance. When the body enjoys pH balance, you experience radiant good health. When the body is not in balance, the disease process begins, resulting in problems ranging from bone loss to premature aging and more. The key to a healthy pH is proper diet, but for a long time, acid-alkaline food guides have included only a small number of foods. Or they did, until now.

The Acid-Alkaline Food Guide is a complete resource for people who want to widen their food choices. The book begins by explaining how the acid-alkaline environment of the body is influenced by foods. It then presents a list of thousands of foods and their acid-alkaline effects. Included are not only single foods, such as fruits and vegetables, but also popular combination and even fast foods, like burgers and fries. In each case, you'll not only discover whether a food is acidifying or alkalizing, but you'll learn the *degree* to which that food affects the body. Informative insets guide you in choosing the food that's right for you.

The first book of its kind, *The Acid-Alkaline Food Guide* will quickly become the resource you turn to at home, in restaurants, and whenever you want to select a food that can help you reach your health and dietary goals.

$7.95 • 208 pages • 4 x 7-inch paperback • ISBN 0-7570-0280-3

NATURAL ALTERNATIVES TO LIPITOR, ZOCOR & OTHER STATIN DRUGS

What to Use and Do to Lower Your Bad Cholesterol

Jay S. Cohen, MD

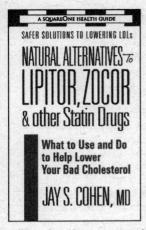

Elevated cholesterol and C-reactive proteins are markers linked to heart attack, stroke, and other cardiovascular disorders. It is estimated that over 100 million Americans—more than a third of our population—suffer from these conditions. To combat these problems, modern science has created a group of drugs known either as statins or as specific commercial drugs, such as Lipitor, Zocor, and Pravachol. While over 20 million people take these medications, the fact is that up to 42 percent experience side effects, and a whopping 60 to 70 percent eventually quit treatment. Fortunately, other options are available. Here, for the first time, is a concise guide that explains the problems caused by statins, and offers easy-to-follow strategies that will allow you to benefit from effective natural alternatives.

Written by a highly qualified researcher and physician, *Natural Alternatives to Lipitor, Zocor & Other Statin Drugs* begins by explaining elevated cholesterol and C-reactive proteins. It then examines how statins work to alleviate these problems, and discusses possible side effects. Finally, the author highlights the most important natural alternatives.

If you have elevated cholesterol and C-reactive proteins, or if you are currently using a statin, *Natural Alternatives to Lipitor, Zocor & Other Statin Drugs* can make a profound difference in the quality of your life.

$7.95 • 160 pages • 4 x 7-inch paperback • ISBN 0-7570-0286-2

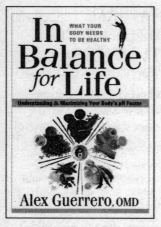

In Balance for Life

Understanding & Maximizing Your Body's pH Factor

Alex Guerrero

The principle of balance is not new. It forms the very foundation of both Eastern and Western philosophies, from Aristotle to Confucius. As it relates to health, it has been around just as long, from the development of traditional Chinese medicine to the treatments used by Hippocrates and Galen. What is new, however, is a scientifically based application that can improve numerous disorders and maximize your health.

Imagine that the human body has an internal mechanism that keeps two basic types of chemicals—acid and alkali—in balance. When your body becomes either too acidic or too alkaline, you become susceptible to a host of disorders. When balance is restored, however, so is your health. In this brilliant book, renowned health expert Alex Guerrero explains how you can become well by restoring your pH balance. The author first describes how you can assess your health, and then provides a fourteen-day diet and a simple program of supplements that will bring your body back into balance. You'll even find a selection of recipes that will tempt your taste buds as you reclaim your health and well-being.

In Balance for Life presents the simple steps you can follow—each and every day—to enjoy boundless vitality and optimal well-being.

$15.95 • 192 Pages • 6 x 9-inch quality paperback • ISBN 0-7570-0264-1

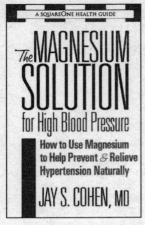

A SQUAREONE HEALTH GUIDE

The MAGNESIUM SOLUTION for High Blood Pressure

How to Use Magnesium to Help Prevent & Relieve Hypertension Naturally

JAY S. COHEN, MD

THE MAGNESIUM SOLUTION FOR HIGH BLOOD PRESSURE

How to Use Magnesium to Prevent & Relieve Hypertension Naturally

Jay S. Cohen, MD

More than 50 million Americans have high blood pressure—a devastating disease that can lead to heart attacks and strokes. Doctors routinely prescribe drugs for this condition, but these medications frequently cause side effects. As a nationally recognized expert on medications and side effects, Dr. Jay S. Cohen wants to make you aware of a safe, natural solution to high blood pressure—the mineral magnesium.

Magnesium is essential for the normal functioning of nerves, muscles, blood vessels, bones, and the heart, yet more than 75% of the population is deficient in it. Dr. Cohen has written *The Magnesium Solution for High Blood Pressure* to provide you and your doctor with all of the information needed to understand why magnesium is essential for helping to prevent and treat high blood pressure. Dr. Cohen explains why magnesium is necessary for normal vascular functioning, how to use magnesium along with hypertension drugs, and the best types of magnesium to use. Most importantly, Dr. Cohen has made the evidence-based research on magnesium's safety and effectiveness highly readable and usable by anyone.

$5.95 • 96 pages • 4 x 7-inch mass paperback • ISBN 0-7570-0255-2

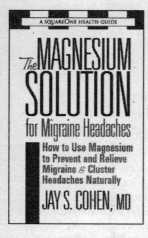

THE MAGNESIUM SOLUTION FOR MIGRAINE HEADACHES

How to Use Magnesium to Prevent and Relieve Migraine & Cluster Headaches Naturally

Jay S. Cohen, MD

More than 30 million people across North America suffer from migraine headaches. Over the years, a number of drugs have been developed to treat migraines, but these treatments don't work for everyone, and come with a high risk of side effects. Fortunately, Dr. Jay S. Cohen has discovered an alternative—magnesium.

This easy-to-understand guide explains what a migraine is, and shows how this supplement can play a key role in preventing and treating migraine headaches. It also describes what type of magnesium works best, and how much magnesium should be taken to prevent or stop migraines. For those who are looking for a safe and effective approach to the prevention and treatment of migraine and cluster headaches, Dr. Cohen prescribes a proven natural remedy in *The Magnesium Solution for Migraine Headaches*.

$5.95 • 96 pages • 4 x 7-inch mass paperback • ISBN 0-7570-0256-0

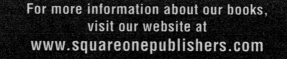